Acts of Kindness
from Your Armchair

Acts of Kindness from Your Armchair

Anita Neilson

AYNI BOOKS

Winchester, UK
Washington, USA

First published by Ayni Books, 2017
Ayni Books is an imprint of John Hunt Publishing Ltd., Laurel House, Station Approach,
Alresford, Hants, SO24 9JH, UK
office1@jhpbooks.net
www.johnhuntpublishing.com
www.ayni-books.com

For distributor details and how to order please visit the 'Ordering' section on our website.

ISBN: 978 1 78535 617 9
978 1 78535 618 6 (ebook)
Library of Congress Control Number: 2016956056

A CIP catalogue record for this book is available from the British Library.

Design: Stuart Davies

Printed and bound by CPI Group (UK) Ltd, Croydon, CR0 4YY, UK

We operate a distinctive and ethical publishing philosophy in all
areas of our business, from our global network of authors to
production and worldwide distribution.

CONTENTS

Acknowledgments

To my husband Paul for his strength and support. To Jenny for spiritual guidance and friendship always. To Amanda, thank you for your amazing typing skills and encouragement. To Kit for unwavering support. Thank you!

Foreword

If you ever thought that your physical circumstances were a barrier to making a positive difference in the world, in this gem of a book Anita Neilson gives practical guidelines on how to change the world from your armchair with thoughts, words and acts of kindness. I found this to be a thought-provoking and very do-able book. Anita leads us along a path from our immediate environment to making changes in how we approach our responsibility to be kind to ourselves, to each other, and to opening our hearts to embrace the whole world.

Anita has walked this path herself and is speaking from her own experiences. When she and I, as work colleagues, became ill with M.E. (Chronic Fatigue Syndrome), we had a choice to lie down to it or to find a way to internally change our experience and to transform into the butterflies that we are: not cocooned, but free to expand and grow beyond our physical limits in any way that we choose.

I have the privilege of knowing Anita as my best friend and confidante. She has never judged harshly and always finds the kindest of ways to support others during their, at times, painful growth and emergence from their own chrysalis. I am delighted to support her first steps in the literary world. *Acts of Kindness from Your Armchair* has the potential to lift you from cocooned and marooned to heart-expansively free. I am proud to wish Anita every success with this wonderful debut book.

Jenny Light
Author of *Living Lightly: A Journey through Chronic Fatigue Syndrome (M.E.)*, Ayni Books

Preface

Acts of Kindness from Your Armchair is an exploration of how the housebound and infirm can live a spiritual life and make a positive, meaningful contribution to the world through acts of kindness and compassion to ourselves, to others, to the natural world and to the environment. The readers' focus is gradually reframed from inward-looking to outward-acting, echoed in a growing realization that we are all reflections of God and each other and therein lies our power.

Why focus on *Acts of Kindness from Your Armchair*? Ill health during the past few years has meant that I am mostly housebound. As a fibromyalgia and M.E. sufferer, I am uniquely placed to write about kindness and compassion from the point of view of those who, for health or other reasons, have to spend the majority of their time at home. A secondary school teacher, until illness hit in 2009, my journey back to health—physically, emotionally, mentally and spiritually—has been long but rewarding (and is still ongoing). Through this time of transition, when moments of social isolation left me feeling unable to contribute, I often asked myself the question: "How can I do acts of kindness from home, from my armchair?" And thus the book was begun.

Interweaving knowledge and techniques from 'traditional' therapies (such as Cognitive Behavioral Therapy (CBT), physiotherapy and mindfulness) with 'alternative and additional' therapies (such as Spiritual Response Therapy (SRT), Reiki, yoga, nutrition and meditation), its overall aim is a desire to share the spiritual knowledge and practical skills gained to date with others.

Acts of Kindness from Your Armchair is not aimed solely at

2

fibromyalgia and M.E. sufferers. Those are merely my personal circumstances. It is written from the unique standpoint of the 'housebound,' those of us who for whatever reason (ill health, disability, responsibility as carers, retirees, parents caring for children, those working from home, among others) find ourselves at home for the best part of the week but wish to make a difference to others' lives through acts of love and kindness.

> *Everybody can be great...because anybody can serve. You don't have to have a college degree to serve. You don't have to make your subject and verb agree to serve. You only need a heart full of grace. A soul generated by love.*
> Martin Luther King Jr

For those with less than perfect health, be that physical, emotional or mental, making a meaningful contribution to society may seem an unattainable goal. Disabilities and mental health issues have in recent years become more mainstream, discussed more openly in public. Much greater billing on television, and other media, of events such as the Paralympics and Invictus Games (for wounded servicemen and -women around the world) contributes to this normalizing and provides encouraging signs to a fairer, more inclusive society.

Acts of Kindness from Your Armchair contributes to this journey. Large-scale, visible acts of kindness are the 'big picture,' if you like. Our acts of kindness are the threads that knit the whole tapestry of the world together: the power within *all* of us regardless of our state of health, or our physical or financial limitations. No apologies should be made for the perceived 'smallness' of our acts, for each of us has a role to play on Earth and all are of equal merit. So, perhaps your 'Armchair' is a wheelchair, your bed or the chair in your study. You are always connected to the world around you and this book shows you how.

Anyone who wants to begin or continue their journey to self-realization through spiritual development will find joy in the pages of this book. It is divided into four parts: Kindness to the Self, Kindness to Others, Kindness to the Animal Kingdom, and Kindness to the Environment. I have not been paid to recommend any websites or products. I simply include the ones which have worked for me personally. There is a wealth of choice out there for you to explore and find what resonates with you.

Writing *Acts of Kindness from Your Armchair* has been a voyage of discovery for me. With hindsight comes recognition that illness was a blessing, allowing me to objectively analyze the person I was; giving me space to discover this new person I have become; and finally blessing me with a faith in the future. I have discovered that as I heal myself through kindness and compassion this helps me to become a kinder person to others—warmer, more compassionate, a better listener, more understanding—facilitating the spread of love that grows in my heart day by day out to others. There is no greater joy than that. I hope you enjoy your own journey.

Anita Neilson

Part I: Kindness to the Self

Introduction

What is kindness? What does it mean to be kind? The Collins English Dictionary defines it as "considerate, friendly and helpful." Kindness is fundamentally about letting love into our hearts so that we can then share it with others. After all, kindness contains the word *kin*, our fellow man.

Acts of Kindness from Your Armchair will teach you to enrich your daily life with thoughts, words and acts of kindness. It will awaken your mind to the possibilities available to you and the power within you, while at the same time providing practical tools and techniques to bring love and kindness to the forefront of your life. The ideas and techniques contained in this book are a *mélange* of all the spiritual and practical knowledge I have gained to date, gleaned from everything which I have read, studied and practiced over the past years and which, crucially, I have found to be useful and beneficial.

The focus of this first part, Kindness to the Self, is on dealing with our inner world in the first instance, learning self-kindness and love. Be assured that we do have the power to change the way we feel, think and act on the inside. The skills learned here may then be expanded outwards to show kindness to others, to the environment and to the natural world.

There are several 'Practices' in the first part of the book. These include: a Cognitive Behavioral Therapy (CBT) practice recognizing and changing patterns of thinking and behavior; a meditation on handing these over to God; a CBT practice on core beliefs and strengths; the power of positive thinking; a mirror-gazing, confidence-boosting activity; keeping a daily journal of gratitude plus acts of love and kindness; a mini-mindfulness meditation to find your place of calm; putting kindness traits into action; a lovely grounding exercise; a solo-tasking mindful check-in; counting your sugar intake; and finally changing from fear-based to love-based emotions for everyday life. Do try the ones which resonate with you, if not all of them. You will gain benefit from them, I promise.

For those of us who spend the majority of our time at home for whatever reason (be that illness, infirmity, work, childcare and so on), feelings of isolation may creep in over time, leading to negative thought-patterns and emotions, which, if allowed to persist, can overwhelm us and affect our ability to make rational decisions. The techniques in this book are designed so that you will notice a subtle shift in your thought-patterns to positive, optimistic and loving—qualities of kindness. They are all chosen from personal experience.

Self-kindness includes facing up to those qualities, bad habits, conditioning and character traits which we may already know are lacking in kindness. This requires honesty and sincerity on our part. Kindness to the self provides us with opportunities for self-improvement and growth. To grow we must face challenges, for if we remain in *stasis* we do not grow. Each of us needs to experience challenges, difficulties and failures in order to really know what success feels like. The ultimate aim for us is to be content and to love ourselves on the inside so that we may positively affect the world around us on the outside with renewed love and kindness.

Chapter 1

Compassionate Self-Analysis

Compassion is the greatest attribute of kindness. It's desirable, if not essential, to learn to have compassion for ourselves first, to strengthen our spiritual core, and then this kindness can pour easily onto others. Compassionate self-analysis entails changing well-established patterns of thinking, old habits of behavior, and replacing them with positive alternatives.

One pattern of behavior which is prevalent in societies of any kind—be they religious, civic, educational, familial and so on—is that of judgment. We judge others in a split second simply from their outer appearance or an action. Yet we know that our physical body is just one of the many layers which make up this person that we are on Earth. We know that behind our physical appearance lies our real self, and that to be the recipient of harsh judgment ourselves is hurtful. We feel it as a punch in the solar plexus, our center of energy in the body. Judgment literally knocks the energy out of us.

For me, judging people began as a piece of childhood fun. My sister and I often engaged in this game—as we saw it—for the self-centeredness of childhood blinds us to the feelings of others. This co-dependence allowed the pattern of behavior to continue unchecked: sitting in church on a Sunday whispering derogatory remarks about others; harshly judging others we saw on television; in fact, in all areas of our lives. This pattern continued into adulthood and became the norm for me as it is for many others.

When we first begin our compassionate self-analysis, our initial emotions can be those of shame and regret at our past behavior and unkindness. But know that when we go through the process of handing our past behaviors over to God/the Universe, we free ourselves of regret. It allows us to view judgment as a learned behavior and to progress to the next step of actively and sincerely choosing to do things differently from now on. A sincere desire to change is essential, however.

Practice 1: Handing over unkind thoughts or habits to God

For the first part of this practice, you will need a pad of paper and a pen, or, if you prefer, a tablet computer or PC. If you find it difficult to write, many tablet computers or smartphones have a microphone icon in the keyboard which allows you to dictate and the computer will automatically convert this to text.

Whichever method you choose, the purpose of this practice is to honestly acknowledge your unkind habits of behavior or thinking. Write each one down. Use the following headings as a guide:

What is the unkind thought/behavior?
When did the thought/behavior start?
What was behind it?
Why did it continue unchecked?
What alternative ways to think or behave can you choose instead?

Start with those habits which come to mind first. Here are some examples to guide you: saying sorry all the time; complaining about pain; making snap judgments of others based on their appearance or actions; a defeatist attitude; grieving for your past self; temper tantrums; impatience with yourself or others; fear of change; talking yourself down and so on. Look at all areas of your life: relationships, profession, leisure, education, spiritual, mental, physical.

Now, for the second part of this practice, sit quietly for a few minutes where you won't be disturbed. Try to slow down your breathing and sit very still. Concentrate on your breathing. Notice how the in-breath feels through your nose and the out-breath from your mouth. Focusing on your breath calms the mind and body, allowing you to access the 'inner you' — the real self, your innate wisdom. Sit like this for a few moments until you feel more relaxed, breathing softly. Now, recall the first behavior habit from your list. Bring up the earliest memory you can of this and try to see yourself in the memory. Imagine how this behavior is hurting yourself or others. Try to analyze the behavior in a detached way and reason in your mind an alternative, less harmful way of dealing with things. Sit with this process in the stillness and acknowledge this past behavior. Notice with the curiosity of an onlooker the emotions this memory stirs within you. Now take a deep breath in, breathe out through your mouth, and as you do, release any regret, guilt, or shame. Affirm out loud that you sincerely choose to do things differently now, and then hand it over to God or the Universe.

As soon as you hand something over to God, fill the space with love. Imagine the love as a bright white light coming in from above your head to rest in your heart. Feel the heat of this light; see it glowing in your mind's eye, filling the space left by the clearing. This unconditional love feels amazing when we allow it prominence. It reminds us that we are an amazing reflection of God. In order for us to be closer to the Creator we need to love ourselves first, and this clearing exercise will go some way towards achieving this. Sit quietly now for a few minutes and enjoy the stillness and peace within.

Practice this gentle self-analysis and compassionate forgiveness regularly, at least once a week, taking each behavior in turn. You will need to revisit these issues in the future, as they will surface again and again until you have dealt with them fully and sincerely. It's so important to rid ourselves of stuck emotions and unwanted habits of behavior, for left unaddressed, these blockages can lead to us becoming 'stuck' on our life path and unable to move forward.

There are many guided meditations available online (either free on YouTube or available as apps to download onto your phone or computer) to help release blockages and encourage feelings of connectedness to others. Please refer to the Further Reading and Multimedia List at the back of the book for my recommendations. Another useful tip is to stick post-it notes up where you will see them regularly throughout the day. Pin one up for each issue you deal with. For example, you may write on it: "I choose to speak kindly of people" or "I let go of regret and shame." It feels good to unburden ourselves of these past behaviors which no longer serve us.

Crystal therapy is an interesting subject which I have only just begun to investigate more fully. Crystals work with the energy meridians and chakras in the body, in a similar way to yoga, tai chi, acupuncture and Reiki, to maintain a state of balance. The chakras are believed to be the energy centers of the body-mind. Whether or not you subscribe to this belief, it is universally understood that our emotional and mental health has an effect on our physical health: put simply, if we are depressed, our bodies 'contract.' This tension has a negative effect on muscles and connective tissue, resulting in us having less physical energy. Conversely, the happier we feel, the 'lighter' we seem to be; our muscles are relaxed and more blood is allowed to flow, resulting in us having more energy. The seven major chakras run in a line from the groin area up to our crown. The heart chakra in particular connects us with our environment and others. Indeed, our breath is shared with the space and the people around us. As our poor behavior choices result from negative thought-patterns, continuing to make poor choices closes off our heart and creates a 'separateness' from others. We become more detached and cannot move forward on our path. To be kind to ourselves, we need to realize that we are not separate but part of the Whole, be that family, neighborhood, society, country, world, universe, God.

I wear a rose quartz crystal pendant which sits at the level of the heart to amplify feelings of connectedness to and love for others. According to Philip Permutt, author of *The Complete Guide to Crystal Chakra Healing* (see Further Reading List), rose quartz is known as the "love stone" and "soothes upsets and emotional wounds." Malachite is also associated with the heart chakra, bringing calm. Crystals may be placed on the site of the chakra on the body as you meditate to release these emotional blockages which are themselves the causes of the learned behaviors and thought-patterns which you wish to relinquish. Alternatively, you can place a crystal inside your clothing or in your pocket as you go about your day and also under your pillow at night.

Even if this therapy does not resonate with you, know that it can do no harm. It's strange that we take science, medicines and traditionally accepted therapies such as counseling, physiotherapy and so on as fact—as proven treatments. Yet we do not do likewise with other therapies with which we are unfamiliar. We seek proof of their efficacy. All we require is faith.

No matter what our issues in life, at times we need the

assistance of an 'expert,' be that a medical doctor, a physio-therapist, a psychological counselor and so on. My chosen experts at present are beyond the field of 'traditional' healthcare. They are a Reiki therapist and a Spiritual Response therapist. I have found both of these therapies to be beneficial, not only to emotional health but to physical and spiritual wellbeing also.

Reiki is a gentle healing for the whole body where the therapist lays his/her hands over, or gently on, parts of the body in turn to release blockages and re-energize. Reiki flows through the affected parts of the energy field and charges them with positive energy. "It raises the vibratory level of the energy field in and around the physical body where the negative thoughts and feelings are attached. This causes the negative energy to break apart and fall away. In so doing, Reiki clears, straightens and heals the energy pathways, thus allowing the life force to flow in a healthy and natural way" (from www.reiki.org). Sometimes you may feel that part of the body buzzing as if an electrical current were being passed through, or you may experience a sensation of warmth or involuntary muscle jerks. Just trust that all is being done for your highest good. At the same time as the therapist is channeling Reiki to me, I inwardly affirm my intention to release any and all emotional or behavioral blockages. A good Reiki therapist may come to you if you are unable to travel. Reiki can do no harm. It is a joyful, effective, loving kindness to yourself which I thoroughly recommend.

Spiritual Response Therapy (SRT) works quite differ-ently from the above energy meridian-based treatments. "The SRT therapist will work to research and clear old past life programmes, vows, blocks and clear karmic records etc using a pendulum and charts" (from www.living-lightly.co.uk), allowing us to progress more smoothly on our life path. The pendulum is used as a means of accessing information not available to our conscious minds from our intuition. This can be anything from analyzing nutritional deficiencies and food allergies, to assessing compatibility of medication, negative interferences, past-life traumas, problems with teeth/mouth, relationship problems with family members and so on. (Please see Further Reading List for more information.) I have received SRT 'clearing' on a few occasions, some in person, others by distance healing, and have felt an almost immediate shift as the problem/energy block has been lifted. This has to be carried out by a trained SRT therapist but is extremely powerful and worthwhile.

Chapter 2

Celebrating Your Good Qualities

You, yourself, as much as anybody in the entire universe, deserve your love and affection.
Siddhartha Gautama (Buddha)

This chapter celebrates you. Remember that this 'you' is composed of many layers, each interwoven with and inter-dependent upon the others: personality type, character traits, body type, childhood conditioning, psychological makeup and so on. Many of us are predisposed to focus on our negative points, and if this is with a view to self-improvement, then that can be a positive thing. However, if this negativity is solely as a means of self-punishment, then it is fruitless. It's much more loving to yourself to recognize and celebrate all the good qualities which you already possess, an abundance of kindness inherent within each of us.

The Buddha reminds us to love ourselves as well as others. He is telling us that we are worthy and that our worth is equal to that of any other man (or woman). Why do we find it so difficult at times to show kindness to ourselves and, more especially, to celebrate our good qualities? Cultural reasons may account for some of this. In some countries or societies, it is viewed as inappropriate to 'boast' about ourselves, as people may believe us to be immodest and elitist. Peer pressure and a desire to be liked/loved lie at the heart of it for others. We want to fit in with the norm, do as everyone else does. For others still, it's generational. You don't 'blow your own trumpet.' Organized religion has played its part too, encouraging humility and a dependence on God for all our goodness (God-ness).

Self-awareness seems to have been rather demonized over the years and used as a means of control over others. Be assured that it is not solely concerned with knowing our 'bad' points but also and especially celebrating our good ones. I reluctantly use the words 'good' and 'bad' here, for I believe everything about us is essentially good. We are worthy. We are good enough and we deserve our love and affection as much as anybody in the entire Universe.

Practice 2: Focus on your positive qualities

Your kindness practice is to note down your good qualities. Do not focus on your physical attractiveness here, for your body is just superficial, a skeleton which we have to allow us to move around in this world. That's not the real you. If you find this task difficult, ask a friend or family member to help you. It is undoubtedly easier to list negative points about yourself, but shyness and modesty have no place here. You have many good qualities.

You may find it helpful to divide your list into four 'strength' areas: physical, emotional, mental and spiritual. Here are some examples to help you get started. Under physical strengths, perhaps you are a hard worker or you take care of your body by exercising. Under emotional strengths, are you a good listener? Perhaps you are even-minded and not prone to emotional highs and lows. In terms of mental strengths, an ability to multitask when required could be added to your list, as could a tenacity in distracting yourself from pain by engaging in a mental activity such as a Sudoku or crossword. Kindness and compassion towards animals, a sense of gratitude for the blessings in your life, and meditating could all be listed under spiritual strengths. As you go through your compassionate self-analysis, and continue with this practice, recognizing your good qualities, you will come to realize that we all put on masks throughout our lives and these masks also change over time. We become the person that we think other people want us to be in life, clothed in the many layers of personality, character, culture, religion and profession.

Write a couple of your good qualities on post-it notes where you will see them regularly as you go about the house. The power of positive thinking is well-established among psychologists, hypnotherapists and self-help authors alike. Positivity diminishes and counteracts any negative thoughts we have which may taint our view of ourselves and prevent us from taking action. For example, if we think we are going to have a bad day, we probably will; if we think we are unable to paint, then this will reduce our motivation to even try and we will always be bad at painting in our minds. Positive thinking does change our outlook on the world. I use it every minute; each time I have a negative thought, I immediately replace it with a positive one. Think the best of yourself— always. Be grateful for all the good qualities which you possess. Love who you are now, accept who you were in the past and don't worry about the person you might become in the future. Further, if you love God, it follows that you have to love yourself because we are all reflections of Him. So, stop hurting yourself and start loving yourself from this day forth, faults and all. It's the ultimate kindness for you.

Practice 3: Mirror-gazing activity

Mirror-gazing is an established meditative practice with some claims of entering altered states of consciousness after prolonged single-pointed focus, gazing at one's reflection. Rest assured you will not be doing that in this instance. The aim of this practice is not to enter a deep meditative state but rather to boost your confidence and self-love in an easy, practical way, to help you see who you really are and to reinforce positive messages about yourself. It has been a comfort to me and effective at lifting my mood. Sit in front of a mirror, or hold a small one up in front of you. (If you prefer, look at a photograph of yourself.) Look into your eyes in the reflection. Breathing softly and slowly, just gaze at your reflection for a few moments. Let your face soften and look into your eyes (or the space between them).

Now, think back to the list you have just written of all your good qualities. Keep your gaze on your reflection in the mirror and speak to yourself with a gentle, loving tone as you would with a friend. Say what you love about yourself. Here is an example of the type of thing you might say: "I love that I am a good listener. I love that I am kind to animals. I love that I am creative." Then finish with "I love that I am." Hold onto the positive feelings which arise from these affirmations for as long as you can and beam this love to your reflection. Do this every day for an instant boost to your self-confidence!

Chapter 3

Less Is More News

Be kind to yourself and reduce your exposure to news via any of the media platforms (mobile phone, computer, radio, television or newspapers). Reducing our exposure to news helps to keep us on a much more positive footing as this conscious detachment from others' slant on world events may prevent us being buffeted by the latter. For those of us who are highly sensitive, these emotional swings can easily drain us of precious energy.

One beneficial way to reduce our exposure to news is by turning off smartphones or tablets, for even five minutes at a time, at regular intervals throughout the day. Switching off your phone when in company enables you to give your full attention to the person(s) spending their time with you and at the same time allows them to feel respected and loved.

A second way to reduce our exposure to news is to desist from watching news bulletins on television. Think back to childhood. For some it was a happy, loving time. For others, childhood unfortunately meant being the recipient of criticism and/or belittlement. This steady drip-drip effect of negativity over time can lead us to believe that these harsh, negative words are truth. But what is truth? Simply someone else's interpretation of an idea. Just because we read or hear something repeatedly, doesn't make it true unless we choose to believe it is so. This drip-drip effect of negativity and fear is also prevalent in news coverage. News organizations are businesses. They want to make a profit and to do so they have to sell news. Therefore, it needs to be as exciting as possible for the consumer. And we, the consumer, want interesting, entertaining news. Positive feel-good stories are lovely for a few minutes to lighten the mood at the end of the bulletin, but the main stories, in order to enhance their appeal and extend their shelf-life, need to heighten anxiety and fear, bring excitement and drama.

Think about the word 'consumer.' We are taking in news as if it were nourishment, feeding all of our senses. Our ego side loves excitement and drama as it makes life more interesting. But this nourishment is short-lived and ultimately leaves us wanting more, feeling dissatisfied. And remember also that news is someone else's view of events, not ours; a part of the truth, yes, but not the whole truth. We need to retrain our senses to be stimulated in a way that will bring us long-term meaningful joy—seeing the beauty in the outline of a tree against a blue sky; hearing our pet snoring at our side; touching a houseplant tenderly as we speak to it, gently encouraging it to grow; smelling dinner cooking in the oven; the feel of freshly laundered sheets and so on. Do yourself a kindness and switch off the news. Know that it's within our power now to take it or leave it.

If you are a traditionalist like me and prefer hard-copy news then positive newspapers are a great alternative, containing positive, life-affirming news stories which will maintain your link with the outside world in a much more beneficial way. Please refer to the Further Reading and Multimedia List at the back of this book for more of my news portal recommendations. We all have the power to make a simple choice. Do we buy our usual newspaper even though we know it is filled with biased, sometimes spiteful coverage of world events? Why immerse ourselves in a deluge of negativity, spite and fear when we can bathe in the lightness of joyful, positive news coverage? I choose the latter. It involves perseverance, however, as we need to read more closely and retrain our senses in order to discover the excitement and drama of these stories.

Absorbing too much sensationalist news coverage opens the gate for those of us who are highly sensitive to be buffeted emotionally by this super-sensory experience. This can have the effect of reinforcing fear and anxiety, exacerbating depression and dis-ease. Many people, especially those of us who are based mostly at home, find it comforting and a source of company to have the television on in the background, yet this continuous consumption is detrimental to our wellbeing and there are much better behavior choices we can choose for ourselves.

Learning not to be buffeted by world events takes effort and continuous practice, electing instead to effect positive change in our world from the inside out. By choosing kindness and compassion, we can lead by example. We can change the part of the world over which we have a little control—the part within and around ourselves. Remember also that for every one act of evil there are thousands of acts of kindness in the world, and that's where our focus should be. Ultimately, how we think impacts on our reality. If we are full of anxiety and fear about world events, then this becomes the reality we create for ourselves—one full of anxiety and fear. Focus instead on positivity, kindness and love. We know that evil is still present and always will be, so long as selfishness, fear, suspicion, greed and jealousy are given free rein. We can detach ourselves from all this and simply choose to focus on the positive. In this way we create the lighter world we desire for ourselves.

There are conflicting views among psychologists and researchers as to the effects of watching violent television programs and movies, and playing extreme video games. Some base their findings on the research in the 1970s by Albert Bandura on social learning. He surmised that children learn through copying. The content of television programs was found to be a factor in increased aggression in children and a decrease in their sensitivity to the pain and suffering of others. Others disagree with this viewpoint. This is the norm in academic circles. Each person holds a strand of the overall truth. My advice is to listen to your intuition. If you feel uneasy watching something 'dark,' such as a documentary about a mass murderer, or a television program immersed in violent acts and nasty, evil behavior, or a soap which buffets the emotions too much, then switch over or switch off. The choice is in your hands.

I know from experience that maintaining an even-mindedness in everything I do and watch has made a significant difference to my positivity and compassion towards others. A different kind of excitement is to be found in programs about the history of art for example, or traveling through the medium of television to far-off, exotic places, full of cultural vibrancy and beauty. Programs whose *raison d'être* seems to be judging others, be they 'documentaries' about people living on benefits or programs making fun of people whom society judges to be 'undateable' and so on, are of no interest to me. Retrain your eyes and ears and spend your media time positively. This is not solely a self-kindness but will also imbue your relationships with others with renewed love and compassion.

There are many positivity blogs, books and daily affirmation sites you can use to help maintain your positive frame of mind (see list at back of those which I have found to be beneficial). Positive affirmations at the start of each morning will nourish your soul far more than negative news ever will. They are a useful and powerful act of kindness to yourself. Start today with this affirmation:

"I choose to spend my media time positively."

Chapter 4

Being Thankful

Are you a glass half-empty or a glass half-full person? I admit to being the former in the past. Youth brings for some a tremendous sense of entitlement and when things don't go according to our plan, we blame others or make excuses. We rarely think that our negative attitudes may be contributing to our failures. Many psychologists believe that we have an inbuilt tendency to notice the bad things in life, the possible threats as we see them. Perhaps this can be traced back to our Stone Age predecessors whose very survival hinged upon their ability to notice threats on the horizon. It does help to explain why many of us hold a negative view of life: the glass half-empty standpoint. At the extremes, those in this group rationalize that because they will never be successful, there is no point in trying.

However, I have seen that for every negative act, every act of disappointment or despair, there are thousands of acts of kindness and love throughout the world. If our focus is solely on the negative aspects—as we perceive them—of life, our vision may become blurred to the good things around the periphery. That's why it's important to give gratitude every day for the blessings in our life. Remember also that when we focus on things which we perceive as a threat, this often triggers the stress response (the 'fight or flight' response) which can be incredibly harmful to our bodies. It produces noradrenaline which floods our system; increases heart rate and pulse; induces feelings of nausea; and causes muscles to tremble and shake in preparation to 'fight' or 'flee.' This is a useful inbuilt genetic program which kicks in in times of extreme danger. However, our stressors/dangers are other people in cars, screaming children, barking dogs, all sorts of things which invoke this hitherto 'emergency' response time and again. If this physiological response is allowed to continue over time, it may damage your health.

It's certainly easier to look on the negative side of life if we have an inbuilt propensity to view the world in this way. It takes a lot more effort on our part to counteract this tendency and focus on the positives, all the blessings in our life. We have to retrain our minds not to take our blessings for granted but to be grateful for them. The following gratitude practice has proved to be very beneficial to my mental health, allowing me to climb out of the well of depression where I saw no glimmer of hope, to sit calmly in the warmth and light of positivity and optimism.

Practice 4: Daily gratitude

Make a note of five things which you are grateful for every morning. If you prefer, say them in your head, but I believe it's beneficial even for a couple of weeks to write them down. This allows you to look back and gain an overview of your thoughts and words. Some people prefer to record their daily gratitude journal onto a tablet computer using the microphone keyboard icon. Do this every morning before rising, at morning coffee break, or some other time to suit you. Be sure to say why you're grateful for the blessing and what difference this makes to your life.

Here are some of the things I am grateful for and why:

- I am grateful for the fact that I work from home and can keep my own hours, as this flexibility is really important to me and gives me a sense of control.
- I am grateful for my dogs, as they get on well together, and are good company for me.

- I am grateful for electricity because it provides an abundance of energy for cooking and heating. In this way I can wake up in a nice warm environment which helps my pain with a lovely hot cup of tea which soothes my soul.
- I am so thankful for my sense of hearing, so that I can listen to the birds at the feeder in the morning. This makes my heart sing.
- I am grateful for my friends as they make me laugh and keep me positive.
- I am thankful for the family into which I was born. My parents instilled diligence and perseverance in me which allowed me to prosper in life, and my siblings are a constant source of friendship for me.

Make your own gratitude list. It may be tempting to allow your ego to intervene in this process, noting down things which it thinks you should be writing down to make your life appear more exciting. But no-one else needs to read this list. No-one will judge you. Simply write down what you're grateful for this day.

If you're thankful for your husband's patience as he cares for you, because this makes your life so much easier, write this. If you're grateful that you live in the middle of a city because you love all the buzz and the noise, write that. List the ones which resonate with you. Everyone's list will be different.

Practice 5: How did I show love and kindness today?
The second practice in this chapter is to note how you showed love and kindness today. I do this at the end of the day, lying in bed. Reviewing your day, remembering what you did, and more especially, in what ways you were loving and kind, is an act of kindness to yourself. It focuses

the mind, enabling you to analyze events and how you made someone else's life better that day. Break this practice up into three sections: kindness to the self; kindness to other people; and kindness to the natural world and the environment. You will read more on how to show kindness to other people and to the natural world in the later parts of the book. However, as you have been working your way through the practices in Chapters 1 through 3 of this part, you will have gleaned many ideas on how to show love and kindness to yourself. Focus on those in the meantime, and as you progress through the book, add into your practice ways in which you show kindness to other people and the natural world.

To help you get started, here are some things which you could include:

- I showed kindness to myself by eating healthy food because I know it helps to keep me strong.
- I showed love and kindness by watching something other than the news. In this way I was more positive, which I know is good for me.
- I showed kindness to myself by meditating on one of my poor behavior choices from the past and handing it over to God.
- I showed kindness to myself by sitting out in the garden for a while, just being with nature. It is so good for the soul: the birds singing, the flowers showing off, the warmth of the sun on my bones, the smell and sounds of grass being mown.
- I smiled at the grocery delivery man and engaged him in a conversation. He showed me a photo of his dog on his phone. That made us both smile!
- I showed kindness to the birds by making sure their feeder was topped up. Otherwise they waste vital

energy flying in only to find there is no food, and I do love to watch them.

- I showed kindness to others by joining in a remote meditation, sending love and positivity to world leaders as they met to discuss a peace plan for a Middle Eastern country which has been ravaged by war for years.

Being thankful is a major way to show love and kindness to ourselves. It also has the added side-effect that our renewed positivity will affect those around us. Even if we don't say anything, they will perceive by our demeanor and outlook that we are much more positive and thankful. So, be kind to yourself. Change negativity, sarcasm, pessimism, lack of motivation, a glass half-empty attitude, to positivity, optimism, compassion, determination, glass always half-full! You will become a better, kinder person if you effect these changes in your life.

Chapter 5

Meditation and Prayer

Meditation is the most beneficial and wonderful act of kindness to the self. Many people may have practiced yoga in the past and found the postures extremely relaxing, not realizing that it was a kind of meditation in motion. Likewise, losing oneself in an activity, going with the flow and not noticing anything else around, is also a form of meditation, in so doing, finding that inner core of stillness and joy. I have practiced meditation for some years now, learning to quieten and relax both body and mind, to allow my spirit, the true self, to come forth. Daily meditation is greatly beneficial to our physical, mental, emotional and spiritual health. Physically relaxing muscles enables us to eliminate stress and lower blood pressure; mentally it quietens the mind, clearing it of the endless (and pointless) chatter of thoughts about the past and future; emotionally we notice our emotions but learn to be influenced more by our intuitive feelings which this stillness of mind and body permits us to access; spiritually, meditation brings us in touch with our spirit, our true self, that spark of the Divine in all of us, and it is from this place that we become closer to God. It also lightens mood, increases contentment, and enhances kindness and compassion in all of us.

When we first begin meditating we may struggle with frustration at being unable to quieten the 'busy' (egoic) part of the mind, the part which likes to be in control at all times, filling our head with thoughts, fears, what ifs—doing anything but meditate. In this case it's beneficial to find a good meditation teacher under whose guidance you will learn to keep the mind busy with either a breathing task, a visualization task or a concentration task, such as gazing at a candle or saying a mantra. Any of these activities keep the egoic mind occupied, allowing the other part of the self, where I believe our soul resides, to come through.

Practice 6: Mini-mindfulness meditation

Try this mini-mindfulness meditation. Sit comfortably in your chair and make sure your legs are slightly apart, soles of the feet resting on the ground, arms resting in your lap, palms facing upwards. Take a few deep breaths, gently bringing your shoulders up to your ears; breathe in through the nose and then release the shoulders down softly and breathe out through the mouth with a long, gentle exhalation. Do this three or four times. Now just sit and be aware of this relaxed, soft breathing. We are going to bring in the senses and concentrate on them to keep the mind busy for a few minutes.

Concentrate on your sense of hearing. What do you hear far away in the distance? Traffic on a busy highway? Perhaps an airplane flying high overhead? Come a bit closer to home—what do you hear outside? Keep coming in closer, this time into the house. What do you hear inside the house, in other rooms, in this room? Keep coming in now, inside your body—what do you hear there? Your stomach rumbling, your heart beating, your pulse? Sit with these sounds and concentrate on any other sounds you hear within your body. When thoughts come into your head—and they will—don't get frustrated, just acknowledge them and send them on their way.

Bring in the sense of touch. What can you feel? What do you feel from the soles of your feet? Tingling? What do you feel from your fingers? How do your clothes feel on your body? What about your physical body—how do your muscles and limbs feel? Do some areas feel softer, more relaxed than others? How does it feel in your body to breathe in and out? Keep focusing on these pleasurable physical sensations. Again when thoughts come in, notice them and send them on their way. Now, what do you see with your eyes closed? Imagine you can see the room you're sitting in. Keep your mind busy by visualizing this in your head. Where are you sitting in the room? Can you see yourself? Try and look at yourself from different angles. Does the room appear light or dark?

Allow the sense of smell to come to the fore. Perhaps you may smell something cooking, or your own perfume? Simply focus on what you can smell for a moment. This is such a lovely time just for you. You don't have to do anything, you don't have to be anywhere, just here, just be here, now. Don't struggle against the silence. Struggle is detrimental to meditation. Furthermore, silence in meditation isn't a threat but rather a comfort, the destination of choice. Wrap yourself up in its peace and know that you are never alone. Meditation brings us closer to God. Even if we are sitting at home by ourselves, we are never alone. I find great comfort in this thought of interconnectedness. Remember that at all times there are many people meditating around the world simultaneously, connecting with each other. There is such a peace in the silence and unity of meditation.

Now be aware of your feet on the floor and your bottom on the seat. Stretch your arms out and open your eyes. How do you feel? Just sit for a moment and think how you feel. Perhaps your muscles will feel warm and fuzzy, your eyes may feel more relaxed, perhaps your mood will feel lightened? I certainly hope so. I recommend that you practice this mini-mindfulness meditation every day when you have a spare five or ten minutes. In fact, make the time each day. It's important to stop and rest and just be, staying in the present, not thinking of the past or the future, not thinking of anything you have to do, just being.

Mindfulness

There are countless other ways to use mindfulness as a kindness to yourself, many of which can be done from home, even from your armchair. The definition of mindfulness is being present, being completely aware of what you're doing in the moment, no thoughts of the past or future to trouble your awareness of the calm center within. Here are some other strategies for mindfulness which you may find useful.

The practice of walking mindfully entails being aware. Aware in the first instance of your pace (are you rushing— if so why?) and slowing down if necessary; aware of your breathing (are you breathing from your upper chest?—this is a sign of stress) and taking some deep breaths from the abdomen to re-energize and feel the air enter your lungs like a soothing balm; aware of what you see, hear and smell around you (what if you were asked to recall all that you had experienced and seen on this walk—could you do it?). Observe this world and your place in it in a new light. Even if you are walking around the house or garden, engaging all your senses in this way enhances the experience of walking and you should return from your walk much more energized and joyful.

Another way to be mindful is to really appreciate what you're eating, rather than just consuming your food at the same time as doing something else and/or as quickly as you can because you're ravenous. Instead, slow down. Take a bite. See how it feels in your mouth. Savor all the different textures and flavors, the heats of all the different spices. Be thankful for the food and for all the people involved in growing and producing it.

You can be mindful when doing chores. Don't rush through them just to get on with the next thing which the ego part of you believes will be more exciting than what you're doing at present. Simply take your time and find joy in doing these tasks. Do them properly and slowly, thinking about what you're doing, noticing things. In effect, you can do *anything* mindfully.

Praying to God

How many of us pray directly to God, I wonder? Is this simply a childhood habit which we discard in adulthood? We may sometimes pray in times of crisis, but I would argue that praying, instead of being a last resort, should be the first thing we do every day. Prayer is not about asking for material possessions as many of us did in childhood but rather asking the Creator to help us *help ourselves*. I know many people think that we don't need God any longer once we start to make our own way in the world. We find excitement in filling our lives with activities, possessions, holidays, careers and so on. I too have sought happiness through material wealth and prestige in my career. I have had these things and more, and yet was unfulfilled and discontent. It can take some time for the penny to drop, for us to realize that what was missing from our lives was God. We didn't see that coming. We were managing just fine, weren't we? Well no, actually, we weren't.

We think short-term excitement in the form of holidays, new cars, filling every moment with exciting activities, drink, drugs and so on will make us happy. It simply makes us want more and more. Ultimately this results in unhappiness, the opposite of what we imagined. This is a really big moment in our lives because it's the start of self-realization. We realize that what we were really searching for was long-term joy, peace and contentment and that we will find these things with God. We understand finally that God is better than all the wonderful distractions on Earth that He has given us. So try to find your space of inner peace, morning and night, and pray to God. Try this:

A prayer to God for our time
God, the Creator, Source of All that Is
May we find on Earth Your heavenly bliss.
We praise You, beloved Father
And follow and trust in Your word.
Sustain us with Your life-force
In this ever-changing world.
Teach us to love others in Your way
Help us to show forgiveness
Each and every day
Guide us and keep us safe
As we journey back to Your domain.
While the veil of delusion is lowered
Like a drawbridge from our eyes:
We praise you, Lord, as we realize
That bliss comes not from this Earth
But from knowing and loving You.

Communication with Angels
There are some who would find praying to God an awkward experience—for many reasons (lack of confidence or an overwhelming feeling of deference, to name just a couple). For them, an acceptable middle ground would be communicating with the Angels. All Angelic beings are non-denominational and non-gender specific. To be able to 'hear' the Angels, we need to detach ourselves from our busy daily activity for a while, and the best way to do this

is through meditation.

Meditation quietens the 'busy' (egoic) mind, home to the ego which likes to be in charge of our life, filling the mind with thoughts and fears of things past and future possibilities. Meditation enables us to access that place of peace within us, the sanctum of inner silence, and from this place, to connect with God, or the Angels if we prefer. Angels can seem to be remote beings, depicted as they are in paintings by the great masters, embodied in churches as statues, mentioned in sacred scriptures. They are ethereal, closer to God. However, be assured that the Angels are also close to us. They can't intervene in our lives, as God has given us free will to make our choices on Earth. Nonetheless, if we ask for their help, the Angels will gladly give it. They often send us repetitive signs, intuitive feelings or thoughts to help us in answer to our prayers, so it's important to be vigilant to these signs. Read the last sentence again and remind yourself to be more aware of these signs in the future.

Through quietening the mind, we tap into the Angelic wisdom and can ask for the strength to face certain things or to help us increase our intuition and so on. There are many books on Angels and Archangels which list their characteristics and what you can pray to them for. My advice is to choose one or two favorites. Mine are Archangel Michael for strength and determination, and Archangel Raphael for healing and to bring love into my heart. (Please see the Further Reading and Multimedia List at the back of the book for my recommendations.)

I do also ask the Angels for help in times of crisis. Know that they will always help if we pray to them at these times. I have had occasions when I have been in intolerable pain and have cried out to the Angels to help me because I simply felt unable to cope on my own. They have come to my aid every time: either by intuitively prompting me to the name of just the right person who will help me; by the phone ringing and the caller being a friend who has been thinking about me and asking how I am; by bringing me comfort in the way of a song which suddenly comes on the radio; by an article on the very next page I turn to in a magazine; or by giving me an intuitive feeling about which medication to take to offer me optimum pain relief and help me to sleep. These are some of the many ways in which Angels have helped me in times of great need. The majority of us are unaware of these signs, but once we know what form they take, we can train ourselves to recognize them and, more importantly, act on them. Certainly, if I receive repetitive messages (either in written form, intuitive feelings, or words which come into my mind etc.) I *always* act on them because these are always help from my higher self (our inner wisdom) and the Angelic realm. To connect with your Angels you can use the mini-mindfulness meditation practice. This will help you find your inner place of peace and from there try praying, try talking to God and the Angels. All that is needed is effort and an open heart.

Meditation and prayer are very comforting, not least because of the realization that we are never alone. Prayer, through meditation, is the ultimate kindness to ourselves, to our Soul. We must always be kind to our Soul and gentle with our chattering ego mind which will quieten down over time, given dedication to daily practice.

Chapter 6

Kind Thoughts, Words and Acts

At this point, let's recap the kindness skills and aptitudes outlined in Chapters 1 to 5 with the aim of evaluating to what extent we have already shown kindness traits in action. Chapter 1 was about acknowledging poor behavior and thought-patterns, then replacing these with positive alternatives. Chapter 2 focused on discovering our good qualities, celebrating and accepting ourselves as we are. In Chapter 3, I recommended making more informed choices to focus on the positives in life, reducing our exposure to negative viewpoints of world events via the media. Chapter 4 was about gratitude, making a positive choice to be thankful for all the blessings we have in our lives rather than complaining about what we don't have. Finally, in Chapter 5, we learned meditation techniques to bring stillness to the chattering mind in order to let our inner peace shine through. It also focused on relearning how to pray.

In this way, through reading these chapters and doing the practices contained therein, we have opened the flood-gates in our heart to increase the flow of the following traits, which are inherent in all of us but often pushed aside by the ego with its 'What's in it for me?' attitude. These traits are: goodwill, benevolence, charity, compassion, generosity, humanity, kindliness, philan-thropy and understanding.

Search in a thesaurus for synonyms of "kindness" and these are some of the definitions you will find. Through an analysis of our behavior and thought-patterns we come to an understanding of, and compassion for, our past choices, together with a determination to make kinder choices from now on. By being proactively thankful for all our blessings this will reawaken goodwill and charity towards those who are not so blessed.

Practice 7: Kindness traits in action

Look again at the kindness traits listed above. Make a note of each one and beside each one write down any events, however small, where you feel you have made progress in embedding these traits of kindness more deeply in yourself. It may be helpful to have two columns as outlined below with some examples:

Goodwill: I noticed when I was judging a friend unfairly and replaced this with a positive thought.

Benevolence: I joined in a prayer for wisdom for world leaders as they met to discuss a way forward for war-torn Syria.

Charity: When entering a competition, I affirmed to myself that I would give some of the winnings to charity.

Compassion: I watched a television program and felt compassion for one of the celebrities who seemed lonely.

Generosity: Upon receiving four small gifts from my sister, I spontaneously offered one each of the gifts to my other sisters.

Humanity: I felt sympathy for people in the world who still have to walk miles to collect water each day. I will no longer waste water.

Kindliness: I played Hunt the Food with the dogs instead of ignoring them to watch

	television.
Philanthropy:	I bought one of a friend's paintings to encourage her in her art.
Understanding:	I put myself in my husband's shoes after I had cajoled him about something he hadn't done and realized that it doesn't feel good to be the recipient of this.

Other examples of how you have shown kindness traits in action could be: perhaps you have thought more charitably of refugees fleeing for their lives; perhaps you became aware that you were about to say something negative about yourself or others and you stopped yourself and instead remained silent; perhaps you hugged a friend who needed emotional support, and so on. Note down the ones which you have experienced. Read this list often, and add to it, and you will be amazed at what kindness your heart is capable of.

Kind thoughts

If a man speaks or acts with an evil thought, pain follows him...if a man speaks or acts with a pure thought, happiness follows him, like a shadow that never leaves him.
Buddha, *The Twin Verses*

Thoughts create our reality

Acts of kindness result from kind *words*, which themselves originate in kind *thoughts*. The Law of Attraction has fascinated many scholars throughout history from the Buddha to Albert Einstein to Christian Larson (*The Optimist's Creed*) and more recently Rhonda Byrne (*The Secret, The Magic*), to name a few. It proposes that our thoughts create our reality, and what we think, say and do will be the reality that we attract back to ourselves at some point. For example, if we think and say that life is unfair, that bad things always happen to us, that we are never lucky and so on, these negative thoughts of lack *are* the reality that we create for ourselves and therefore we *will* always think of ourselves as a victim in life because it doesn't go the way we want it to. These thoughts lead us to negative emotional patterns where our lack of success—as we see it—may result in us experiencing bitterness and discontent.

Be assured that bad things don't happen to you. Things happen. To us all. Don't take it personally. By changing our thoughts and how we react to life's challenges (which after all are opportunities for us to grow), we create a happier life for ourselves, full of optimism and joy.

The concept that thoughts create our reality is widely accepted in spiritual circles and is also backed up by medical practices today. Cognitive Behavioral Therapy (CBT) analyzes our actions and how they arise from thoughts. These actions arise from inner core beliefs about ourselves. CBT can help people discover what their core beliefs are and which strategies to adopt to counteract and eventually change them. Someone whose core belief is "I'm not good enough" could become very self-critical in their thoughts and words. They may think themselves a burden, needy or stupid and may often voice these thoughts. This negativity can then lead to feelings of sadness and hopelessness. With the support of a CBT therapist, we can learn that it is beneficial to think of compassionate alternatives to challenge anxiety and negative thoughts. This gradually leads to much improved mood and motivation. We are retraining ourselves to think more positively and attract a better reality for ourselves. Instead of adopting the victim mentality of: "I will fail, so I'm not going to try," we would say for example: "What is the worst that can happen?" or "It might be fun!"

So, be kind. Notice when you are being negative about yourself, acknowledge it when it happens, and immediately change the thoughts or words to something positive. Keep practicing this and it will eventually become a new automatic mode of behavior.

Don't compare yourself with others

If you compare yourself with others you may become vain and bitter,
for always there will be greater and lesser persons than yourself.
Enjoy your achievements as well as your plans.
Max Ehrmann, *Desiderata*

It's futile. We live in an aspirational world. We get caught up on the treadwheel of comparison, wanting what our friends have, envying what our neighbors have, pedaling faster each day to try and obtain these things. Our mind is full of 'if onlys.' If only I was 50 pounds lighter, I'd be happy. If only I had that new car, I'd be happy. If only I had a good job, I'd be happy, and so on. Yes, we should do our very best to improve our lot in life but not in order to *be* like someone else, for you know that there will always be someone else with more. Turn your focus inward to your own life and find happiness there.

Love your work

Always try to think positively about your work. Remember to be thankful that you have employment and never be ashamed of your job. Not everyone is meant to be a leader of industry. Not everyone wants to have this role. Try to adopt a positive attitude to your work. If you are unhappy at work, look within yourself first. What is the real root of the unhappiness? What steps can you take to change this situation? We are all capable of being of great service to the world.

Kind words

Stop complaining

Many of us who suffer from chronic pain get into the habit of moaning about it, making exertion noises when we rise, grieving for the person we used to be and so on. But if we cry wolf too often, people learn to disregard our complaints. Moaning about pain can be seductive for the complainer as it brings us attention and sympathy for a little while. However, eventually one sees the light dim in others' eyes as they struggle to counter the constant negativity. Accepting our life as it is, pain and all, is a big step towards leading a more spiritual life, one of kindness to ourselves and others. Acceptance doesn't mean doing nothing to help ourselves, but rather accepting that things are as they are and deciding rationally what we can then do to help ourselves. It is pointless and harmful to complain about aspects of our health or other things over which we have no control, such as the weather or others' feelings. And how exhausting it also is for the recipient to hear these complaints! Ask yourself if your complaints are draining others of their vital energy. If so, commit to changing this habit to a more positive one.

Speak your truth

Another way to be kind to ourselves in the words that we use is to speak our truth. Being ourselves by always being authentic but kind. If we don't say what we really feel then we are diminishing ourselves, we are not being the person we should be. We all put on masks to please or appease others to some degree. Don't be afraid to say what you feel, give your opinion, or disagree with others, yet do it kindly to avoid upsetting them in so doing. Find ways to speak your truth gently.

Here are some other ways to be kind to ourselves by the way that we speak:

Speak kindly of yourself first of all. Don't demean yourself with your words. Pull yourself out of self-victimization. Don't stop trying because you think you will never succeed.

Always look on the bright side, always focus on the positive, always strive to do better.

Speak kindly of others. Don't pre-judge people by something you have read in a newspaper or seen on television. Further, analyze the source of your derogatory comments. Is it jealousy? This is not a good use of your energy, and remember that what you send out into the world in terms of your thoughts and words is what you attract back to you. So if you are judging someone you can be sure that someone somewhere is judging you.

Also, if someone you are in conversation with is judging another person don't react or join in with them. Stay silent and let that silence convey that you will not be feeding their negativity. If you can't stay silent, turn the conversation around immediately and say something positive instead about the person.

One way to speak kindly of others is to join a meditation or prayer group. This can be a physical group of people or it could be joining an online community. There are many spiritual magazines that have online communities, which often make arrangements to meditate or pray at the same time on a particular day. Meditating as part of a group, a community, is such a powerful thing to be part of. It brings peace and calm to us personally as well as increasing the strength of goodwill being imparted to others. If this is of interest to you, you can also download meditation apps onto your smartphone and see at a glance or a touch of a button how many other people are meditating at the same time as you around the world. (Please see the Further Reading and Multimedia List at the back of the book for more details.) Group meditation is so uplifting and motivating. Know that we *can* change our world through kind thoughts and words in meditation and prayer. If you are relatively mobile, you can also think about joining a more formal prayer group of people coming together to pray for and send love and kindness to others who are in need.

Kind actions

At the risk of sermonizing, firstly, in terms of kind actions to yourself, don't over-indulge, trying to find comfort or satisfaction in excess of any kind, be it exercise, food, drink, drugs or the pursuit of material goods. These things don't fill the space that we all feel within us. They may afford brief moments of excitement but these are short-lived and ultimately leave us wanting more. No, the space within us exists because we have forgotten who we really are and why we're here. Meditation, spiritual reading and practices can help us rediscover ourselves and God. For my part, I have found the joy and inner contentment which I sought elsewhere throughout my life but which eluded me. Here are some more ideas of how to show kindness to yourself through your actions:

Allow yourself to have fun every day. Especially if we are at home for the better part of the week for whatever reason, it can become the norm for some of us to focus on the negatives, on what we don't have, rather than to count our blessings. If we are in pain, our pain can overwhelm us and that's why it's good to have a little fun every day. Having fun is a distraction, and in times of greatest pain doing something that distracts us from it, even for a short while, can help considerably. It could be baking a cake, watching something silly on television, listening to a funny audiobook, whatever resonates with you in order to have fun. If you are in company, ask people to tell you a joke, or you tell one. Do some craftwork, knitting, painting; find an activity which is fun, easy and distracting for you.

Secondly, I believe it's important to rediscover our inner child. Expectations change as we grow up through teenage years and into adulthood. It becomes ever more clear that we are expected to assume a mask of professionalism, that we must take our jobs seriously and we must not fool around and be childlike. There seem to be so many things we must not do to conform to society's expectations of us. Reconnecting with our inner child is vital as that's where the more authentic part of us resides—in the part which experiences joy in all of life. So be kind to yourself and do things which remind you of your childhood, and don't mind what other people think of you: wear a silly hat, hand out lollipops to delivery people, play football in the garden with your dogs, sing, make paper flowers, put on silly voices in public and so on. Life wasn't meant to be taken so seriously.

The best way to find yourself is to lose yourself in the service of others.
Mahatma Gandhi

Thirdly, it's important to accept help from others. This is a quid-pro-quo arrangement as on the one hand we get the help we need to do a certain task, and on the other hand we are helping that person to do an act of kindness for us. In effect, as the above quotation says, we are helping ourselves *and* them to become better people, to grow spiritually, by being of service to others.

Next, try to do some gentle exercise every day. If you are chair-bound, seek advice from your doctor or other medical professional and if you can, do some very gentle movements such as you would find in yoga or tai chi. Start off with just a few minutes and very gradually over weeks increase the time and level of effort. There are many good examples of beginner's yoga on YouTube. Exercise keeps the body awake and stops us deteriorating further, so this is a vital, positive kindness to ourselves.

Lastly, get out in nature, even if it's just out onto your balcony or garden. Feel the sun on your bones, watch the birds. If you have trees nearby, notice them: see how the leaves flicker, how the branches gently bow in the wind. Trees are wonderful, so majestic. They teach us much through their resilience and strength. If you can get out near trees then do so.

Practice 8: Grounding meditation

While you are out on your balcony or in the garden try this practice, grounding down into the Earth. Being grounded boosts our energy, decreases stress and facilitates finding the inner peace and silence within us. If you want to, take off your shoes and socks so that your bare feet connect with the ground. Now concentrate on your breathing. Slowly and softly breathe in through your nose, breathing from the abdomen, then out through your mouth. Continue this circular breathing six or more times until you feel more relaxed.

Now imagine that there are roots coming from your toes down into the ground. Let these roots descend and spread outwards under the soil, going further and further down through the rock, down to the very center of the Earth. Here, visualize an enormous ball of light at the center of the planet. This is providing energy to everything. Let your roots touch the bright white light and feel some of the energy coming from it. Visualize in your mind's eye pulling the light up through your roots. See if you can feel the warmth and tingling in your toes as the energy comes up through the ground and into your body.

Feel the tingle in your toes and pull the white light further up through your legs, up into your body and then into your heart. Feel the energy resting there and permeating throughout your whole body. Now you are grounded to the Earth. Sit for a few minutes and enjoy this feeling of connectedness. If you do this practice every day, the tingling feeling in your toes may eventually feel like an electric charge. This is simply your connection to the Earth strengthening, a reminder to us that we are all in essence made of energy. This is a great way to show kindness to yourself by boosting your energy. Your roots going down into the planet are like the cable which we plug into the wall to recharge our mobile phones. In exactly the same way, we are recharging from the Earth.

Solo-tasking

This scene may be familiar to many of you. A woman goes about her day at home. She puts the kettle on to make a cup of tea, as she does so noticing that she needs to order tea bags, so she walks over to the shopping list on the fridge and writes this on it. The pencil is blunt; she crosses to the kitchen drawer and starts rummaging around for the sharpener. Meanwhile the kettle is slowly coming to the boil. Sharpening the pencil she puts the shavings in the bin just as her phone beeps; she takes it out and has a look at the text. As she glances up, she notices that there are a few dishes which need to be put into the dishwasher; this is her next task, all the while glancing at the tumble dryer and thinking, "I need to check that later to see if the clothes are dry." The kettle has now come to the boil. The woman washes her hands and notices that the soap dispenser is low. "I need to order more," she thinks to herself, so now here she is back at the shopping list at the fridge. Passing the worktop she notices the tea bag in the cup and remembers this was the original purpose of coming into the kitchen a few minutes earlier. She had wanted to make herself a cup of tea. She puts the kettle on to come to the boil again and this time stands and waits, finally pouring herself the cup of tea. Does this sound familiar? What has she been doing for the last three minutes—multitasking or overloading her brain?

Multitasking can trigger anxiety because we are thinking about too many tasks at the one time and not really achieving any one very satisfactorily. On the other hand when we do one task at a time we get 'into the zone,' that feeling of deep concentration and absorption, and we achieve a lovely feeling of satisfaction and fulfilment when we finish the task. In effect we lose track of time, we experience 'going with the flow.' What we are really doing is completing a task mindfully, fully absorbed in all the details.

Practice 9: Solo-tasking

Your practice is to catch yourself multitasking when you don't need to be. Don't become frustrated with yourself. Just recognize it, be aware and choose to slow down. Choose to do one task more thoughtfully. Some of us with perfectionist natures are proud of how well we multitask. We haven't recognized yet that it's our ego pushing us to achieve more, to work faster and better than all others. It's simply a learned habit of behavior. Concentrate instead on one thing at a time so that you don't overload your brain. Do this kindness to yourself: don't multitask all day.

Chapter 7

Healthy Eating

Healthier choices

For some of us for whom the greater part of the day is spent at home, isolation, boredom or loneliness can often lead to poor choices in what we eat. If like me you have a sweet tooth, then cakes and biscuits become your comfort and friend. For others it's equally calorie-laden treats such as cheese and chocolate. All food provides the body with energy. However, some foods have lighter energy than others and feed our overall wellbeing. These are unprocessed foods, fruits, vegetables, grains, pulses. We recognize when we eat them that they are nourishing our soul as well as our body, don't we?

Further, we know in our hearts that too much of one food group is not ideal for optimum health. The aim is to create balance in what we eat just as we create balance in our emotional and spiritual health. This can mean finding healthier, but no less moreish, alternatives to the foods we crave. This can be a fun challenge, a treasure hunt if you like! In my case, there are several brands of raw cold-pressed (i.e. not cooked) fruit and nut bars and nibbles on the market these days which are delicious *and* good for you. I nibble on one of these bars when I feel a sweet-tooth moment and can highly recommend them. And actually, the less sugar we eat, the less we crave it. For the cheese-lovers among us, why not try the many different varieties of humus or non-dairy cheese for your protein fix, which are also healthier heart choices. Lastly, if chocolate is your nemesis, try melting just two squares of dark or milk chocolate to dip a couple of plain biscuits into, a delicious and healthier way to satisfy a chocolate craving.

Added sugar in food is becoming a big problem nowadays. It contributes to obesity, type-2 diabetes and heart disease. I urge you as a kindness to yourself to always look at the ingredients when you buy food. The best advice is to be informed. Sugar has other names such as glucose, fructose, corn syrup and so on, and the nearer the top of the ingredients list these appear, the greater the sugar content. This is becoming such a problem that the World Health Organization now recommends that we only consume six teaspoons of sugar a day, just 25 grams.

Practice 10: Sugar tally

Do a tally in your head or on some paper of how much sugar you consume just with tea, coffee, fizzy drinks, sweet treats, breakfast cereal etc. (and that's without the additional hidden sugar in convenience foods which you may be eating for lunch and dinner). The amount of grams or teaspoons of sugar which we consume in a typical day can be staggering. If your total is much more than 25 grams don't be alarmed. You're certainly not alone in this. Accept that you consume too much sugar and make a positive choice to change. It's time now to be kind to yourself.

Our bodies are a wonderful gift and one which many of us take for granted. Just think, the body does everything we ask of it over the many years we inhabit it. It is pushed to the limits physically, mentally and emotionally; we subject it to many different stressors; we overfill it with unhealthy food, drink, drugs and so on. We take from it continuously. Why don't we choose now to start giving back, to nurture the body as we ought to? Indulge in our favorite foods by all means, but do we need to over-indulge? Eating is one of the great pleasures on Earth, that's true. However, emotional eating is not a healthy way to address our problems. It's just a temporary sticking plaster. There's no need for any feelings of shame or regret if we over-indulge in food, just a recognition of a bad habit and a promise to ourselves to make more informed, healthier choices in future.

Some people find cooking problematic, either due to physical impairment or problems with memory and so on. Realistically, convenience foods are a necessity. In this case, when food shopping, choose the healthiest versions of soups and ready meals that you can afford and be thankful that you have the money.

Giving up the foods that we crave, even temporarily, can be turned into a charitable act for the good of others. In January each year my husband and I each give up the thing we crave the most. I give up sugary biscuits, cakes and sweets, and he gives up alcohol. At the end of the month we tot up how much we would have spent on these items and donate the money to a charity of our choice. Not only have we been showing kindness to our bodies but we have also given something back to our community.

Time-savers

Until about a year ago I was doggedly determined to make all meals from scratch, my rationale being a desire to eat more healthily for the good of my body. That's an honorable intention. In reality though, I was struggling with my ego which wanted (and always will want) to be in control of all aspects of my life. I was exacerbating my pain and fatigue by stubbornly persisting in cooking, and this inevitably led to long periods of exhaustion. Further, cooking itself was no longer the pleasure that it once was; it had become a chore to be over and done with as quickly as possible.

This struggle between my ego wanting life to be the way

it wanted it to be, and life actually being the way it was and is, was causing me to experience unhappiness and frustration as well as physical pain and fatigue. Then one day I decided to accept that I was no longer able to cook a big meal. In truth, none of us is the person we once were. I decided to stop fighting and accept. That's not to say I surrendered. I just lowered my expectations, which for a person with perfectionist tendencies is not an easy thing to do.

So now I have discovered the joys of time-savers which allow me a middle ground with some element of control over which ingredients I use in preparing much simplified meals. Pre-prepared vegetables, frozen vegetables, tins of mixed beans and lentils, chopped tomatoes, low-sugar pasta sauces, fresh soups—I make sure I have a ready store of all of these foods. This middle ground doesn't entail slaving at a stove for hours in order to eat healthily, but rather 'going with the flow.' Who cares if you use pre-prepared vegetables? If cooking is difficult for you, let go of your ego, find a middle ground and be kind to yourself. Simplify meals during the week and cook at the weekends only if you have help. Remember that convenience foods are not the enemy if you are careful about salt and sugar content and don't eat them all the time.

Vegetarianism

I became vegetarian for health reasons—a fellow fibromyalgia sufferer recommended it as she had noticed a marked reduction in pain after she stopped eating meat. I have to admit, having been vegetarian for a couple of years now, I have not noticed any great reduction in pain. Neither have I missed eating meat. In truth I had been struggling for a few years leading up to that point with ethical concerns over the welfare of animals reared for meat. Further, I don't believe it was a coincidence that this person prompted me at the right time to take the next step for me which was giving up meat altogether. Coincidences are synchronicities—a nudge from the Divine, if you like—which remind us that we have something to learn from every person who crosses our path. Therefore I have continued with vegetarianism and am slowly progressing towards veganism. It can make us more creative in thinking about food, in menu planning and in a willingness to try new things.

Chapter 8

Choose Love

Many of us on our spiritual journey learn about the concept of duality of life, encompassing such examples as we perceive on Earth: night and day, light and dark, good and evil, the movement of tides in and out, the change in seasons to opposites and so on. In simple terms, duality is about opposing thoughts, emotions, deeds and words. Yet within this duality there is only one relative truth, for night is an absence of day, dark is an absence of light, evil is an absence of goodness and so on. Further, every emotion we have is either fear-based (for example, anger, envy, sorrow, hatred, insecurity, greed) or love-based (for example, compassion, understanding, acceptance, goodwill). Fear is simply an absence of love and originates from the ego side of us which fills our minds with comparisons, suspicions and dissatisfaction. Love comes from our true selves, and by choosing love we choose not to be identified with our ego but with our true self which will bring us more joy and contentment than the ego ever would.

Most of us, until we awaken and realize that we have a choice, live the greater part of our lives in fear. There can be many reasons for this. A need for acceptance by others increases feelings of insecurity and anxiety which plague us. Worrying unnecessarily about not being good enough to live up to our own high perfectionist ideals. Fear of failure and of being humiliated in front of others contributes to our reluctance to try new things. There are, I'm sure, many more examples you can recall from your own life living in fear. How freeing it is now to understand this choice that we have between love and fear and to let go of the fear! For my part, I choose to live differently in this new stage of my life. I choose to live from love in everything I do. When meditating each morning, I ask that everything I think, say and do that day will be based on love, goodwill and kindness. This obviously doesn't happen overnight. However, when I catch myself thinking or feeling negatively, the joy is that I am now aware of doing so and can immediately change to a positive alternative. The more we become aware of fear-based thoughts, emotions, words and deeds and change them to love-based alternatives, the more automatic this will become in our lives. We are retraining ourselves to choose a different way of being and it takes practice and resilience not to give up when we fall back into fear-based being, but to dust ourselves off and keep trying.

Here are some examples of how you can move from fear-based to love-based, positive courses of thought and action in your daily life. The examples arise from my experiences.

Contempt to compassion

Change thoughts of contempt to feelings of compassion. I remember laughing at an ageing pop star who was singing on television as his facelift had given him a surreal mask-like appearance and his mouth could hardly move when he sang. My initial reaction was contempt, a negative, fear-based emotion. However, I quickly realized my unkindness and with this realization compassion returned. For kindness is always there within us, although hidden behind the negative, fear-based, selfish ego. Compassion enabled me to sympathize with this man. He worked in the entertainment industry and would, like many in his situation, doubtless feel pressure to look good at all times and at all ages. Seeing the situation from his point of view, had he felt such a tremendous need to have to undergo painful surgery to his face in order to have the acceptance of his peers? Probably. If so, then he also was living in fear and should be shown compassion, not contempt.

Greed to generosity

Another example, which is simpler but no less important, is greed becoming generosity. In the past I have always baked cakes but then guarded them jealously, not really wanting others to eat them, if I were honest. They were 'my creations' and I was attached to them, wanting them to last as long as possible, holding them close, not recognizing firstly that this was greed and secondly that this greed was a lack of generosity. I realize with hindsight that I hadn't been baking as a kindness to others (as I had told myself) but rather as a means of boosting my ego. And so now when I bake I give the cakes to my husband to distribute to his work colleagues or I take them to friends to share. It's the act of baking for others which is more important than the end result. Changing the focus from ourselves to others brings love back to the fore.

Worry to joy

A third example is when we choose to replace worry with joy. I remember years ago feeling distraught when my mother was diagnosed with Alzheimer's. I worried when she couldn't remember my name; I worried when she had to move to a nursing home. I was making myself ill with grief and worry and yet this was something over which none of us had any control. My sister told me: "Don't worry and grieve anymore for the mother you once had. Just take joy in visiting with a sweet old lady who relishes company." This wisdom spoke to my inner intuition and I made the shift from fear-based worry to love-based joy. I simply experienced joy and happiness in this new person she had become.

Practice 11: Love-based emotions

In this practice, firstly, think of examples of opposing emotions (such as those listed in the first few lines of this chapter), analyze them and evaluate how you can change your initial negative reaction to a situation or person and replace it with an alternative positive one. For example, can you think of a time when you had thoughts of malice towards someone? Analyze this event. How could you change those thoughts or emotions to thoughts of kindness? Put yourself in the other person's shoes; try to see the situation from their point of view. Secondly, think of a situation where you were suspicious of someone; now change that to acceptance, and so on. Anxiety would become going with the flow, jealousy would be replaced with love and goodwill, sadness would become joy, fear would become love.

If you live your life repeating the same pattern over and over again then you are not alive anymore. To die alive is to take risks.
Paulo Coelho

Taking risks

The above quotation from Paulo Coelho, author of *The Alchemist*, is an idea echoed by many psychologists around the world. They recognize that we need to step outside of our comfort zone to try something a little scary in order that we can grow as people. As an ex-teacher I know that we can learn much through failure and subsequent analysis, adapting and trying again until we are successful in our endeavor.

Before you can come out of your comfort zone to try

something a little scary you need to know what your comfort zone is, for it is different for each of us. Ask yourself, what are your self-imposed limitations: physically, mentally and emotionally? Are these realistic? Are they still relevant? Now is the time to push those boundaries a little more every day, every week. For example, at first you could try something new with hobbies: if you have mobility limitations but like to do crosswords, try different types of puzzle—Sudoku, logic problems, word squares. Secondly, change the order of your routine: if you usually walk in the morning, then try walking in the afternoon, or walk a different route. Next, if you know that you are the person who talks most in conversations, try being a good and attentive listener instead. If someone you know is deaf or originates from another country, why not learn a few words in either sign language or their native spoken language? They will really appreciate the effort that you made.

Crystal healing

You can work with crystals to balance and heal any of the chakras in the body. (Please refer to the Further Reading and Multimedia List at the back of the book for more information on crystal healing.) The base chakra (located at the bottom of the sacrum) is associated with strength, change, security, endings and new beginnings, and connects us to the Earth. Use a red jasper crystal directly on the chakra, meditate with it, carry it with you or put it under your pillow at night. This will help to remove anxiety and stress and enable you take advantage of all that life has to offer. And/or concentrate on the heart chakra (located in the center of the chest) which is our center of love and compassion and use a rose quartz crystal in the same way as above. This will ease fear-based emotions and help you see the beauty in everyone and everything.

* * *

All of these acts of kindness can be achieved from the comfort of your own home, from your own armchair. So let the walls of your world fall away around you. Stop living in fear and live in love. We are all part of the one world and what we think, say or do affects all others around us. So make sure your words, thoughts and deeds are positive and love-based.

In Parts II, III and IV of this book we will explore how your growing kindness to others and the natural world will change your life forever.

Part II: Kindness to Others

Introduction

The shift from selfishness to selflessness is a joyous one. The more we can disregard the ego part of us with its incessant wants and comparisons—which only induce anxiety in us—the more we are in touch with our true selves, enabling our innate kindness to blossom.

When we are at peace within ourselves, we see the world, everyone and everything in it in a different, truer light. We see beauty in the simple things; we delight in others' joy; we begin to see our interconnectedness more clearly. It is at this point that a willingness to serve others arises spontaneously.

This section of the book will provide you with many ideas on how you can serve others selflessly with no thought of reward for yourself by being and showing kindness to all, *and* you can do these easily from home. Don't allow your home to be merely a place of safety from the outside world. This is living in fear and is not a kindness to yourself. We are all part of the Whole (world) outside any man-made walls, be they physical or emotional, and we each have a part to play in the Whole.

The examples in Part II (Chapters 9–12) arise from my personal experience and will provide you with copious ideas on how to be kind to others. These include: letting people be who they are: learning life's lessons; our interconnectedness; curtain twitching; inspiring others; nurturing friendships; acts of kindness in person and online; everyone is equal; getting informed; and sharing our good fortune and resources (money, time, goodwill etc.).

Chapter 9

Let People Be Who They Are

The beginning of love is to let those we love be perfectly themselves and not twist them to fit our own image, otherwise we love only the reflection of ourselves we find in them.
Thomas Merton

I believe one of the reasons we are here on Earth is to learn compassion for others. The opposite of compassion is judgment. There are many ways in which we judge others—from their outward appearance, from their words or actions, from their cultural differences and so on. Our preference is to try to fit these 'disparate' others to our own image, to conform to *our* way of doing things. We want people with whom we disagree, or whom we see as different from ourselves, to live their lives the way *we* would choose to live it.

This approach is rooted in fear. Fear of anyone who is different. How do we manage this fear? By trying to control others. For example, I have a learned behavior, going back to childhood, of trying to control people. I remember playing with my friends as a young child and in my memory it is always I who made up the rules for the game which I wanted to play. I can see the pattern clearly now in retrospect. Later in adulthood I controlled people by being moody, a type of soft bullying if you like. This is equally rooted in fear, an attempt to control others to force them to do things our way because we believe that our way is the right way and any other way is wrong and therefore we should fear it. When we are rooted in fear, we see things in black and white. We are controlled by our ego and its fears and desires and this doesn't make us happy.

It's uncomfortable for us all to look back and realize that we didn't love others for who they were, faults and all. On the other hand, selfishness is a natural stage in childhood and so we shouldn't be too hard on ourselves for this past behavior. But by trying to control others, know that we are not respecting them or loving them. Further, those we try to control the most tend to be our nearest and dearest—loved ones, partners, husbands, wives, children, close friends. And all too often a partnership or marriage descends into a competition, both sides vying for victory, attempting to make the other person change to fit their image, to fit their way, and this is where problems result. Inflexibility soon becomes intolerance if left unchecked. Intolerance can lead to hatred and this can lead to breakdown in marriage or any relationship.

Look again at this scenario and see its tendrils spread throughout society and the world. People become intolerant of their neighbors, of their neighboring country, of people of different religions, people in different countries, rich people, poor people, anyone who's different. Intolerance rises quickly from the smoldering embers of judgment where our mindset has become so rigid in believing that 'our way is the best way' and 'everyone else is wrong.'

This is because we are steeped in believing that we are all separate, but this is not the case. We are all interconnected. We all have our role to play on Earth and we each depend on others playing their role to the best of their ability. We are all part of the Oneness of life. We try to control others through fear in a futile attempt to be master of the small part of the world around us. Life becomes much calmer when we can let go of trying to control, and trust that God works through us, having faith that every-thing will be as it should be. The good *and* the bad, for everything that happens in life is an opportunity for us to learn something, should we grasp it.

Those of us who find ourselves at home for the best part of the week may share a learned habit of curtain twitching. This is an example of trying to be master of the small part of the world around us, judging and attempting to control others. This may be the man looking out of his window disapprovingly at young children as they interact with the horses in the field opposite. He sees them make 'bad' choices, prodding them with twigs or bunches of grass. His body may amplify his feelings of unease and disapproval with tics, fidgets, increased heart rate and anger rising like an angry serpent. They are just being children, curious, learning, making mistakes. It may be the woman who hears a crowd of 'rowdy' people approaching along her street. She judges them as something to be feared only to discover that they are a group of teenagers litter-picking. They are just being teenagers, loud but kind.

Can curtain twitching be stopped? Yes, just like any learned habit. These poor habits of behavior can't be stopped overnight though. We have to put in regular efforts to relinquish them to God, replacing them with more positive behaviors. And after all, who are we to decree what is right and what is wrong among human beings? We are all created equally. Let them be, let people be who they are, not who you think it would be better that they were. Children especially need to learn how to interact with the world, just as we all had to learn. We all make mistakes and we hopefully learn how to make wiser and more informed choices as a consequence.

Never try to compel others to change; leave them free to change naturally and orderly because they want to; and they will want to when they find that your change was worthwhile. Christian D. Larson, *Mastery of Self*

A lovely act of kindness to others is to inspire them to be more positive by our words and actions. We humans are programmed to believe what we see with our eyes first before anything else. Who among us has not judged another on the basis of a cursory glance at their outward appearance? When we learn to access the innate kindness within us, we may feel compelled to wish to spread our joy, to tell others how they can be changed for the better. This comes from a place of love (unless it is our ego feeling superior, something we must watch out for). Unfortunately our attempts to communicate this joy often come across as sermonizing or patronizing, telling others what they should do (as we see it), and therefore may result in the opposite of the desired effect.

Inspire others

Simply being who we are and using all the techniques from Part I of this book will positively change our demeanor, attitude and actions. By living our lives differently our inner peace will shine out and be an inspiration to others. They will observe a happier, more contented, kinder, more understanding you. Some will dismiss this as a passing thought; others may be intrigued and inspired, wishing to understand how this change has come about in us and how they can adopt some of the strategies to improve their lives.

So remember to keep practicing the ideas and techniques in this book every day. Start at breakfast time and do your gratitude list in your head or in a journal for that day: things, people, skills, anything and everything that you are grateful for. Gratitude negates the feelings of lack which the ego tries to immerse our thoughts in during the day. Gratitude maintains our link with inner peace and love, from where kindness springs forth. It is equally important at the end of the day to do our "How did I show love and kindness?" practice, analyzing our thoughts, words and acts of love and kindness. Meditation is essential to maintain our link with our true self, ideally twice a day, if not once a day at a suitable time, or first thing in the morning and in the evening. When we are meditating and we reach that state of stillness where our mind is quiet, it is then that we can pray for other people, think of others and shine our love out to them.

Whatever we are doing during the day, do a mindful check-in and observe the body and what it is experiencing. Are we rushing through a task and feeling stressed or contracted? Do we feel a knot in our stomach or solar plexus? Is our mind thinking of the past or the future? All of these are amber indicators. This is our true self reminding us to do things mindfully, slowly and deliberately, not rushing, just experiencing, being present.

Always try to think of others before you speak or act; turn off the news and read positive news instead. All of these things will have an impact in your life but also in the lives of those around you. They will see a great difference in you and you will be inspiring some of them to want to be more positive and kind themselves.

Nurture your friendships

Some of us find it difficult to form and maintain lasting friendships. There are many reasons for this, either because of a lack of confidence, an overpowering sense of competitiveness or a fear of rejection, to name but a few. Whether we have one friend or many, friendships like any other relationship need to be nurtured. Give a friend a hug when you see him or her; tell your friends what they mean to you. If you find it difficult to say it face to face, send them an email or a text. It's all right to use loving language with friends; don't be embarrassed about it.

Also, bring to mind a friend whose character and personality traits you admire and think how you could seek to enhance those traits in yourself, to enable you to become a better friend to them as well.

Chapter 10

We Are All Reflections of God

The truth is that I am eternal, I am never born and never die,
although I am the Lord of all who lives in every creature.
The Bhagavad Gita

The focus of this chapter is the realization that we are all created equal in the world. At the same time each of us is a unique reflection of God. During meditation, when we reach that place of inner stillness, try this practice to reinforce this sense of interconnectedness. Send out love and light from your heart center to your nearest and dearest, to your family, then to your neighbors, and especially to those from whom you feel a separateness; keep expanding the love outward to encompass your town, your country, the whole planet. Visualize the planet from above, reach around the back to the dark side of the planet with your mind and visualize both hands unbuttoning it. Now smooth out the surface of the planet as you would a precious piece of fabric or tapestry. Know that God is the Creator of this tapestry and that he has used the same raw materials to construct this wonderful planet that we live on. Any artist uses the same raw materials to create each part of a painting—although some parts are larger and feature in the foreground, some are smaller and are assigned to the background, and different colors are used throughout—and so all the elements which make up the painting are separate yet combine together to become the Whole. If one or more elements were taken out, the painting would not be complete. The separate parts of the painting, or tapestry, have a symbiotic relationship to maintain the unity of the Whole.

The Earth is God's tapestry. We are programmed and conditioned to believe that we are all different and to fear that which is different, but in reality we have many more similarities than differences: each of us is living a life on Earth with all the experiences that entails; each of us faces challenges in order to grow; each of us is lost and trying to find meaning in life and our way back to the Creator, whatever name we give Him. We are all made from the same raw materials, and part of our life on Earth is to realize that we too have a symbiotic relationship which enables the unity of the whole planet to be maintained. Why do we fear that which is different? If we are working as One, is it not better to embrace difference and delight in it? Wouldn't it be a tedious world if we were all the same? If we looked the same, thought the same, uttered the same words? Everyone is unique; that's amazing, isn't it? Everyone has their own beliefs, their own truth to speak. Their truth is not wrong because it differs from yours. It's just another part of the Whole truth if you like. We each have a different perspective on the truth, and yet all perspectives are right and true.

This calls to mind the Parable of the Blind Men and the Elephant as told by the Buddha to his monks who had been quarreling among themselves and could not agree on an issue. Briefly, the parable relates how a king brought together all the blind men in his kingdom and instructed his man to show the elephant to the blind men, each of whom felt a different part of the animal. They then argued among themselves as to what an elephant was, based on their individual experience of it. The moral of the story is that we need to see all sides of an issue and keep an open mind to be able to form a more complete and accurate view of reality.

Everyone you meet, whether you resonate with them (like or feel a connection to) or not, is a reflection of God. In the Gospel of Luke, chapter 6, verse 31, Jesus says: "Do to others as you would have them do to you." This, like so many other messages from Jesus which may have been misunderstood at the time, rings true today. Treat others as you would have them treat you. Further, as it says in the quotation at the top of this chapter from the Bhagavad Gita, even if we never actually see the original God the Creator on Earth, everything that is and everyone we meet is a reflection of God, including ourselves. It is an important act of kindness therefore to desist from judging others out of fear of that which is different.

Equally, the Law of Attraction affirms that what you give out into the world is what you will attract back to you. The Gospel of Luke elaborates on this concept further on in chapter 6: "But love your enemies, do good, and lend, expecting nothing in return. Your reward will be great." Therefore, immediately you have a judgmental thought of others, put yourself in their shoes and change your thought to a positive one. It is widely accepted in spiritual circles that we choose our parents and family before we are born, together with the circumstances in which we are born and some lessons to be learned in this lifetime. So if someone chooses to be born to parents with emotional or social problems or into a family in poverty or drug addiction, should we not be applauding that person spiritually rather than condemning them on the basis of what we observe on the surface, namely, they are poor or they don't have our standards, or they are an addict? Ask yourself, could you live in a family situation like that? Bless others for their choices and the path they have chosen in life if it's a particularly difficult one. Remember also this wonderful quote:

The tongue, like a sharp knife, kills without drawing blood.
The Buddha

One really important way to show kindness to others is to stop trying to win arguments. This stems from the feeling we have that we are all different, that we are all separate and that we should fear this difference or separateness because it's a threat to us. These fearful emotions arise from the thoughts of our egoic mind which wants to be in control of our life. To be at peace, we need to accept that we are all essentially the same.

All of us have differences of opinion with others, sometimes many times during a day. When the ego is involved, differences of opinion often escalate into arguments; each conversation becomes a competition, an attempt to try and dominate another person. Dominating others is the opposite of kindness. By forcing your opinion on someone, you drain them of their vital energy in order to make yourself feel superior or right. You diminish them. Sometimes this may even be evident in a physical manifestation. Their shoulders may drop, their head may nod in concession, their breathing may become shallow and so on. And yes, you may feel good temporarily with this 'victory,' but celebrations are short-lived and often replaced with regret, that hard-knot feeling in your solar plexus.

What would happen if you let others have the last word? If you agreed to disagree? If you found a compromise? Who is really winning if you are trying to impose your will on someone else? Why is your way the right way and theirs wrong? Who are you to say that your opinion, your will, is the only way? Aren't we all created equal? The other person's point of view is just another part of the 'truth' after all. No-one has all the answers, and part of our purpose on Earth is to learn from each other through understanding.

These concepts of separateness and difference are an illusion.

All the great spiritual teachers and formalized religions through the ages have concurred on the idea of treating others as you would like to be treated. Do not try to impose your will on others, as you will also be diminishing yourself, stunting your spiritual growth. Socrates believed that if you harm someone else you harm your soul. And yet we repeatedly seek to protect ourselves physically and emotionally through trying to impose our will on others, so that we don't get hurt. This is the underlying fear behind arguments. This shutting down or battening down the hatches is a false sense of security, however. It leads to greater harm in the long run, spiritually, emotionally and physically.

Do yourself and others a great kindness and accept that this other person has a different point of view. That's it. You both have different parts of the whole truth and neither of you is completely right or completely wrong. The twentieth-century yogi, Paramahansa Yogananda, said that maintaining a calm emotional state gives us the skills to overcome life's challenges (paraphrased). If you feel you or the other person is becoming angry, walk away; go and be calm somewhere else. It doesn't matter if they think they have won — there is no winning. Adopt this new strategy from now on and if even one person starts to notice this change in your behavior then you have done them a kindness as well.

Another good way to show kindness to others and simultaneously allay your own irrational fears about differences is to learn about them. For some this may be an intolerance and fear of particular groups of people such as teenagers, foreigners, the landed gentry, or people of other religions (particularly those featured in frenzied media reporting). Be informed. Learn about them; immerse yourself in their world to an extent. This may make you much more tolerant of them and realize that you have many more similarities than differences. Go online, do some research, speak to other people, try to find out what similarities you have and this may lead you to re-examine your attitudes and become more tolerant of and compassionate towards them.

Chapter 11

Kindness in Person and Online

Let's remind ourselves of the principal meaning of kindness, that of allowing love into our hearts in order to share it with others, our kin. Keeping the attributes of kindness in mind as we go about our day will serve as a useful *aide-memoire* in helping us to help others. Some of these attributes include: goodwill, generosity, humanity, charity, philanthropy and compassion. Their common denominator is of course love. When meditating in the morning or doing our gratitude practice, end with a prayer to the Creator that everything we think, say or do that day shall be based on love; all our thoughts, words and acts shall come from a place of kindness.

The message being conveyed through reading this book and working through all the practices is that kindness shines through all of us in the smallest of acts. Know that this kindness will have a positive effect both on ourselves and also on the world around us and those who inhabit that space. Love and kindness are attractive to others. Our spontaneous acts of kindness may ignite the spark of kindness in them, for they will wish to share in the joy and peace so evident in us as a consequence of our kindness to others.

This book is packed full of ideas which have worked for me in recent years. I have to stress that I didn't try everything all at once! Lessons are learned from the actions and words of others, through trial and error, and through an increased trust in the guidance of our intuition, for it will quietly provide guidance in the background if we are open to listening. Our intuition will always guide us to a path that's for our highest good.

Section A: Kindness in person or by telephone

Treating people how we would like to be treated is an essential part of kindness. Here are some suggestions on how to put this tenet into practice:

Always look people in the eye—any visitor to your home, be that for a social visit, a delivery or someone providing a service to you. This may seem unnecessary to mention, and yet how often do we not take the time to look people in the eye? This is a poor, learned habit of behavior which may have its foundation in laziness or some other reason, but which may be received as disrespect. Keep in mind that communication is a two-way process and that what we intend to convey is not necessarily the message which is received. Of course, some may say we live in stressful times and people are very busy. And yet, if we don't connect through our eyes, we become disconnected, we sever our link with our 'kin.' Meeting others' gaze is a simple, yet powerful act of kindness which can have an enormous cumulative effect.

Bless and thank people for the service which they have carried out for you, either in person or by phone, for their service is an act of kindness to others. Thank the delivery person for being so gentle with the groceries or a package, for example. Buy a Christmas bottle for people you appreciate, the postman for instance; or chocolates for the staff of the local pharmacy who deliver prescriptions to your home (what a great service that is!) to make them smile and show how much you appreciate them.

Do not take your anger or frustration out on a customer service agent. He or she is an employee, carrying out their job to provide a decent life for themselves and their families. So thank them for being kind and patient with you. Speak to them calmly and respectfully. If you find yourself becoming angry, pause and regroup. Put yourself in their place. Would you be able to cope with the stress of having people's anger directed at you all day at work?

Compliment someone on a skill or aptitude. This may be a family member or a waiter, cleaner, dog walker, cat sitter, whoever makes a difference to others. Be aware, however, that a compliment suffixed by a comparison with yourself negates this act of kindness. For example, if you say "Oh you do that so well. I used to be able to do that but I can't now," what you are really saying is "Poor me. I can't do that any longer. Give me your sympathy." Demanding others' sympathy or attention actually diminishes their life energy. It is very important therefore to be honest and sincere in your compliments.

Spontaneity is best when it comes to giving compliments. I remember a time recently when a friend and I stood and watched a learner driver reversing the car around the corner at the side of my home. When he had finished, my friend and I both spontaneously applauded him. This made both the learner driver and the instructor smile. Further, it brought broad smiles to our faces. It feels good to make other people smile.

Divine Father,
Teach me the value of kindness to others
Show me the merit of loving my neighbor
Help me to serve with no thought of reward
These things I pray from this day forward.
Anita Neilson

Tell someone why they are important to you or why you admire them.

Smile genuinely at people. A true smile comes from the

eyes as much as it does the mouth! Treat others as you would like to be treated. Wouldn't it feel lovely if someone gave you a big smile completely out of the blue? A smile is infectious, beaming love and kindness from one person to another.

Be a good listener and show understanding to people. Often when we have conversations we can end up monopolizing the conversation, being the ones always talking and relating stories and events. Some people like to be the center of attention, but it's much more of a kindness to others to curtail this part of you. Practice being the one who asks questions and actively listens to the answers, with no nodding or attempts to interject with your contributions.

Make people feel welcome in your home.

Always keep in mind your motivation in helping others. Our apparent altruism and selflessness is tempered by that part in us all which likes to be thanked and covets the praise for helping others and being kind. Your motivation should be selfless, an act of being kind because it's the right thing to do, because each act of kindness leads to a better world, because we are effecting positive change in the world around us.

* * *

Putting our words into action makes it much more likely that we will inspire others by our deeds rather than by preaching. Have you thought of giving up sweets, biscuits or alcohol for a month, then donating what you would have spent on these in that month to charity? This takes a lot of resilience but is so worthwhile when you make your donation at the end of the month. You can do this from home, from your armchair, with ease.

If someone does you a service, an act of kindness of any

sort, don't complain about the way they do it, or try to interfere. This is the egoic part of your mind trying to exert control. Remember that we all have different ways of doing things, different views, distinct opinions, but not one of us has all the answers to the questions life poses us. We rely on each other. Cede control graciously and give thanks for this act of kindness.

I read recently of one woman who tries to instill in her children an appreciation for how blessed and fortunate they are in life and to appreciate that there are children who are not so fortunate. It's now a tradition of theirs that for every toy they receive for Christmas, they give one to charity. This is such a special act of kindness for a child to do; a selfless act with no thought of reward.

Section B: Kindness online or by post

Always try to leave good reviews and feedback for online companies. This is especially important for smaller companies as this spreading of goodwill is vital in helping them grow their business. This small act of kindness only takes a few minutes of your time but can make a great deal of difference to the online company.

Give your support to online campaigns which resonate with you. This could range from spreading the word via your online contacts, to signing up to the online petition to ensure an issue is debated in your parliament or house of representatives, and so on. Some television programs focus on particular issues, such as excessive sugar in food and drinks, and have a text number or website URL for you to sign up your support. One such program was successful in having a sugar tax debated and subsequently passed by the UK parliament. This online campaign network is growing in strength and becoming a potent force for change in attitudes and laws. Your support, given easily from your own home, means that you are effecting positive change on a national level. That's amazing, isn't it?

Donate to fundraising online or on television. Large-scale fundraising campaigns, such as Children In Need (in the UK), rely on the viewer enjoying the entertainment which has been laid on for them, in order to reap the benefit of generous donations to worthy causes. I have often watched these programs in the past and not thought to donate. Now, I feel so blessed and grateful that I have the money and want to make a difference that the least I can do is to make a donation to the charity via text. Donate what you can afford. It all changes people's lives.

If you take a good photograph why not let someone else know that you are thinking of them and send or share the photo with them via your phone or tablet computer. This short message will delight the recipient and is a simple, loving act of kindness from your heart.

The Law of Attraction

One of the Laws of the Universe, the Law of Attraction, simply put, enables us to attract into our lives that which we focus on. In short, our thoughts create our reality, perhaps not immediately but at some point in the future. For example, if you are sending out thoughts of love and goodwill to others, then these will come back to you, from someone at some time in the future. Here is a simple example to demonstrate the power of this Law: I took a photograph of a posy of flowers which I had gathered from the garden and shared the photo with a couple of friends. I received an almost immediate return message from one friend who said, "It's like a floral prayer all on its own!" This made me smile with joy. I hadn't sent the photograph in order to receive praise back from others. I just wanted to share something beautiful with friends. And yet the joy had come bouncing back at me via text. It was lovely.

The Law of Attraction has links with Luke's Gospel in the Bible (see Luke chapter 6, verses 27–38). This is the part where Jesus is talking about treating others as you would like to be treated yourself. He states: "If you love those who love you, what credit is that to you? For even sinners love those who love them." It is easy to love people we feel connected to, isn't it? It takes steadfastness to maintain a positive frame of mind about others from whom we feel a separation. And yet the advice of Jesus is: "Do not judge, and you will not be judged; do not condemn, and you will not be condemned. Forgive, and you will be forgiven." This is the Law of Attraction in practice!

Sponsorship. There are so many sponsorship schemes available online if this is of interest to you, such as sponsoring a child in an African village to enable him/her to attend school; sponsoring a conservation program for endangered species; or sponsoring the Hunger Project to end world hunger, and many more.

Send a card or a surprise gift to someone. This simple act of kindness reconnects them to you, letting them know that they are loved and that you are thinking of them. If you are unable to get out to a post office, you may be able to set up an online postage account with your domestic mail service (Royal Mail in the UK) and print off a postage label from home. Ask someone to pop it in a post box for you.

* * *

This list is obviously not all-encompassing. These are my suggestions and you will find a wealth of ideas on online websites to do with kindness, positivity or happiness.

(Please refer to the Further Reading and Multimedia List for my suggestions as a starting point.)

Chapter 12

Share Your Good Fortune

We can be fortunate in many ways in life—financially, spiritually, being blessed with intelligence, being blessed with children, being loved by others and so on. The first thing we can all share with others is our kind thoughts: thinking positively about people, sending love and goodwill to others during meditation or at any time throughout the day. The daily practice of meditation may include a focus on one of the attributes of kindness in order to improve this attribute in ourselves for the good of others. It could be our generosity of spirit and thoughts; it may be our sense of humanity towards others; or perhaps a growing awareness of how we can be charitable to others, not solely in our thoughts but also in our words and deeds. This chapter deals with how we can share the good fortune (mostly, but not exclusively financial) which we have in life with others. Read the suggestions below and try the ones which resonate with you.

Donate!

- Donate money to a cause which resonates with you.
- Donate time. (Can you tutor? Help someone to read? Spend time with an elderly relative?)
- Donate baby clothes you no longer need to younger members of the family or to local charity shops.
- Collect scrap paper or cans to raise funds for local schools.
- Donate books to your local charity shop or library.
- Donate food. For instance, if you order food online, order a few more cans or packets of staple foods to

donate to food banks. Also, give a thought to the fact that if you can afford to buy yourself better quality food, why would you spend less money on food to donate to others? Are they lesser than you? No, of course not. Buy the same quality food for them as you would for yourself.

Organ donation

Of course the ultimate donation is organ donation. Some of us may feel queasy about this, but know that this (the body) isn't who we are. It is merely a shell, a structure which allows us to move about on this planet. Who we are is the Soul, a spiritual non-corporeal being which discards the body when it has no further use of it. There are many people who have not given birth to new life in this lifetime. What better way, then, to end your life than to give life to another! Have the conversation with your family and friends. Tell them your wishes, and register online or by telephone to be an organ donor. In this way, you may give someone else a second chance to live a fuller life. This is a real test of your sense of humanity and connectedness to others.

Give back for the greater good

Always give back. If we only take from others in life, we stifle our own spiritual growth. Some people are very generous to their family and loved ones. However, this is easy to do, isn't it? More difficult is giving back to those from whom we feel separate or different. If you have been fortunate financially in life, then do think of ways in which you can give back to those in need. This does not necessarily have to be financial. It may be giving back in terms of your time, giving advice or mentoring others.

Make it your choice this year to give 1% of your income

to charity. Some of us live on low wages or pensions, while some of us are more fortunate. Know that we all can afford to give 1% of our income. Take a moment to work out what this figure would be on a monthly basis and you will see that it is not an onerous amount. If everyone were to commit to giving 1% of their income, this would fund a tremendous amount of charitable projects, both at home or abroad. Start the ball rolling in your part of the world; lead by example and start giving.

Work on your philanthropy, another attribute of kindness. To do this, try crowdfunding. It's fun. This is a new, online phenomenon where entrepreneurial, often start-up, businesses ask for funding via a crowdfunding website. This could be the young farmer raising a specific amount to buy cows, or a forestry project abroad raising an amount to buy farm machinery, or the www.positive news.org website placing a crowdfunding appeal to enable them to continue producing the website into the future. This is an especially kind way to share your good fortune in a small or big way, since traditional banks are loath to lend so freely in the aftermath of the financial crash of 2008.

Pray for others during meditation. Sending love and light to those with specific illnesses or a generalized prayer for all who need love and support in the world is giving back, sharing your light with others. Remember not to focus on the illness but to visualize them as well and happy. This kindness spreads love, goodwill and compassion across the globe. And remember the Law of Attraction: what you focus on increases so make sure what you focus on is based in positivity and kindness.

Buy 'fair trade' products if you can. The fair-trade movement gives fairer prices and improved conditions to small producers in developing countries around the globe.

Their products (mostly commodities such as sugar, tea, coffee, cotton, chocolate, crafts and so on) are slightly more expensive for us, the end user. However, by buying products from smaller fair-trade producers we are playing a small part in promoting sustainable development in those countries and redistributing some of the wealth away from large-scale, traditional producers. In the long run, this may be cheaper than providing charitable aid to those countries. Do as I do. Give thanks for the money you have and give something back to others less fortunate.

Social enterprise

Social enterprise cafés or businesses are springing up in towns across the UK. These are in the main not-for-profit organizations. They train and employ people who may have been deemed 'unemployable' by traditional employers: perhaps victims of drug abuse; perhaps vulnerable and unable to live independent lives up to this point. These social enterprises demonstrate many of the attributes of kindness; they give back to the community, providing employment; teaching soft skills such as how to relate to people, and aspects of personal hygiene and table manners etc. Our support of a social enterprise café could range from suggesting that you eat there the next time you go to lunch instead of the usual high street (solely for profit?) restaurant; to offering financial or mentoring support. Get informed if this resonates with you. Read up on your local social enterprise(s) with a view to formulating in your mind how you might support them and give something back to others less fortunate.

Part III: Kindness to the Animal Kingdom

Introduction

In reading this book, we are all undertaking a journey of realization of our *interconnectedness*. We began with the Self in Part I where I outlined many skills and practices which you may choose to adopt to improve your own capacity for kindness. This is why we are here on Earth, to experience what it is to be human in order that we might improve aspects of our soul and find our way back to Source.

Part II expanded on this sense of interconnection by outlining ways to think of others first, before ourselves, and not to think of any reward we might gain in showing kindness to others, but simply to be kind because it is the right thing to do. Remember that we are part of the one world. We are all parts of God's creation. We are all parts of God, the Creator. Think about that. No-one or no-thing is lesser or greater than the other.

In Part III, this is expanded further to encompass our interconnectedness with the animal world. Many of us profess our love for animals and a desire to protect them, but poaching and hunting continue unchallenged, for example. If we don't see it happening in our part of the world, is it rendered somehow more acceptable in our eyes? We each need to ask ourselves, in a sincere and honest manner, if we want to change our learned habits of behavior towards animals. What is our motivation for change? Peer approval? Financial gain? Because our heart tells us it is the right thing to do?

This part of the book provides ideas on how to rethink our learned beliefs and attitudes towards the animal kingdom. It is a nudge, if you like, for we all need someone to nudge us along onto the next part of our exciting life's adventure. Think back for a moment to people who have been in your life only briefly. In retrospect can you now recognize that they nudged you in some way? For example, perhaps they made you redundant, perhaps they taught you about anger, or opened your eyes to your strengths in some way? This event then nudged you onto the next part of your life. These nudges can often be unpleasant but they are always worth it in the long run, for we learn through the challenges in our life just as we do from the good things.

So how can we be kind to the animal world from our armchair? Part III (Chapters 13 and 14) inspires us to go forward henceforth with a renewed spirit of 'giving back' because it's the right thing to do—spreading love and kindness to all living beings. You will learn about such things as: animal intelligence and what it teaches us; showing kindness to all animals; buying cruelty-free products; and the concept of *Ahimsa*.

Chapter 13

Making Good Choices

Each of us is on the Earth to carry out the functions of the form we have taken. A cat is a cat; a whale is a whale; a wasp is a wasp. They have no choice in the matter of how they behave. Simply being that animal is their *raison d'être*. Humans have higher brain function. We make choices every second of every day. These can either advance us in our quest to be the best human being we can be, or they can hold us back, tethered to a lower level of selfish existence.

Humans possess higher brain function, yet animals still retain many qualities which we aspire to but have lost or tend to ignore—a reliance on instinct, a sense of interdependence for our survival, a respect for differences, and a resilience and steadfastness in our daily lives. Our innate sense of superiority over the rest of the animal kingdom has unfortunately developed into disrespect for our animal friends, resulting in poor, learned attitudes and behaviors towards them. We have killed animals out of fear of difference (who among us has not squashed a spider with a newspaper?) and for entertainment (hunting, cock-fighting etc.). We use products tested on animals, disregarding the pain they have suffered in service to us.

Yet, each time we think of harming an animal, know that we harm ourselves, for all species on Earth are interconnected to ensure the survival of the planet, of the Whole. Where would whales be without plankton? How would birds survive without worms, or polar bears without seals? Each of us has a distinct, yet connected, role to play in life. As humans we need to make the shift from viewing animals as pests or a food source to seeing them as the amazing gifts from the Creator that they are. This is especially true for those animals which we deem to be ugly, dangerous or a nuisance. Our opinions are not to be relied upon too heavily as they are tiny threads of part-truth, ever-changing with our emotions. Instead, we should trust our instincts and intuition.

Other animals have much to teach us. Elephants, for example, possess great emotional intelligence and can show empathy and grief. Also look at how they form tight-knit social groups and fervently defend their young. Dogs vary in intelligence depending on the breed; however, they do respond well in general to human training and have adapted their natural responses as wild animals to be able to live with us. My dogs show me unconditional love; I also learn from them how to take delight in the simple things— living in the now, having fun, sharing affection. Whales communicate with each other and coordinate their activities in groups, working together for the good of the whole pod. There are countless more examples from nature for us to learn from. Even the smallest animals can teach us. Look at how ants coordinate in groups to build nests and hunt for food. I wonder what the animal kingdom would think of us? How would they view us living increasingly solitary lives, littering the planet with the detritus of everyday life, or polluting the rivers and seas? They would see us take and not give back or nurture the planet in return.

So let's look at some simple ways in which we can all be kinder to animals from our own homes, from our armchair.

Choose positive media choices

There are many television programs or films which portray animals as vicious killing-machines, preying on innocent animals further down the food chain. They are and they are not. They are simply carrying out the functions of the form they have taken on Earth to the best of their abilities, be that an anaconda, a hawk or a bee. Don't watch sensationalist programs or films about animals. These just perpetuate the sense of fear and 'separateness' among us and are just one person's view of reality in any case. Choose instead to watch gentle nature programs, of which there are many, which show the beauty of the animal kingdom.

Further, make a positive choice to not just watch but also act to protect our animals. In the UK, the BBC runs a fantastic series of *Springwatch*, *Autumnwatch* and *Winterwatch* programs which include Citizen Science (taking part in bird counts, surveys of animal spotting in various parts of the country and much more). These programs are accompanied by a fantastic, informative website (please see Further Reading and Multimedia List at the back of the book for more details). Step out of your comfort zone and read about an animal of which you are afraid. It may help to allay your fears somewhat.

Make wise consumer choices

Our consumer choices directly affect the animal kingdom. Plastic bags not only pose a danger to babies but they also do damage to our marine mammals, causing death and injury to thousands of seabirds and mammals through swallowing and entanglement. Swallowing plastic can suffocate them or lead to a false sense of satiety, resulting in starvation. If we are unaware of these facts, buying products in plastic bags seems harmless, our right as consumers. Yet the evidence has been mounting for years and is now irrefutable. We must take a proactive decision to do what we can to protect the animals on our planet.

There are hopeful, positive chinks appearing in our armor of imperviousness: beach clean-ups; supermarkets charging for plastic bags; consumers carrying their own reusable bags; and plastic being recycled by more local authorities, of which my local council recycling center is one. Plastics are easily recycled, melted down and made into bottles and trays, damp-proof membrane, polyester fleece clothing and duvet fillings. So, do these acts of kindness to the animal kingdom:

- Always put plastics in the correct recycling bin. This small effort on our part will improve the quality of life and survival of many species in the animal kingdom.
- Carry your own bags with you when you go out.
- Order vegetables in your online grocery shop to come unpackaged, or give instructions for them to be placed in a paper bag.
- Choose cleaning products which don't contain microbeads (this topic will be discussed more fully in Chapter 18).

Buying products not tested on animals

We all like to uphold the tenet of treating others as we would like to be treated ourselves. Yet, there is a certain bliss in ignorance. What we don't know won't hurt us, yes? The aim of this section of the book is not to try to shock you with statistics and gory details of cruelty caused to animals through testing. There is plenty of material out there for you to read, but I would caution you to read from different sources, including independent ones if possible with no vested interest on either side of the arguments. Do this kindness: get informed. Read up on products; research which ones have been tested on animals.

Once you are better informed, it is then up to you how you proceed. You have to make a personal choice whether you want to continue to use products which you know are tested on animals. Is it a price worth paying for you personally? There are many websites now offering cruelty-free products, from cosmetics to cleaning fluids. (See the Further Reading and Multimedia List for my recommendations.)

I've only recently informed myself of unsavory practices in the dairy industry and have made the decision that I will find dairy-free alternatives wherever I can, such as rice milk, coconut cream, soya cream, and sunflower spread instead of butter. These are all readily available from supermarkets and online. If I cannot find dairy-free alternatives, I choose to consume products from organic farms where standards of animal welfare are much higher.

Chapter 14

Ahimsa

The Sanskrit word *Ahimsa* translates as "cause no injury, do no harm, non-violence to all living beings." The concept in Jainism, Hinduism and Buddhism centers around the tenet that all living beings have the spark of the divine spiritual energy within them, and that if we harm another living being, we harm ourselves. I believe this is a kinder way to live our lives, being and showing kindness to all others, and I have sought to express this throughout the book. Incorporate *Ahimsa* into your daily life. Radiate your love and kindness out to others. Your light will brighten their spark and yours. Here are some more ideas on how to show kindness to the animals in your part of the world.

Feed the birds

Set up a feeder in your garden, balcony or shared yard, and prepare yourself for the joys of bird-watching from home. Once you have a bird feeder the stage is set for viewing snippets of animal life which you may otherwise have missed. Take, for example, the scene of parent birds feeding young fledglings balancing unsteadily on the tray below the feeders, the parents then returning time and again in order to feed their unconfident offspring; or the tiny field mouse sneaking out from under the decking to forage a peanut. Wonderful!

If this is of interest to you, do some homework beforehand. Ask friends or relations for advice; the internet is always a good source of information for what type of food is best for which particular birds. Remember, if you can't physically replenish the feeders, ask for help. Is there someone else who could do this kindness for you? Don't see problems; think of how these can be solved. Asking for help, remember, is a great kindness to yourself and others. Feeding the birds helps to protect vulnerable species and will fill you with joy to sit and watch life unfold around the feeder. You will soon want to buy a bird book to identify your visitors and perhaps even binoculars!

Show kindness to all animals

Fear often drives humans into 'fight, flight or freeze' when confronted by the object of their fear, be that a spider, a wasp, or a mouse. However, the Universe has a way of nudging us to face up to our fears, and so it presents us with opportunities again and again to do just that, in the hope that we will learn a different, wiser way of dealing with our fear. I have been afraid of spiders since childhood and often killed them with a newspaper. Spiders have been appearing on a regular basis in my life until I ordered a spider catcher from a company on the internet. This sucks up the spider into a tube for it to be safely deposited outside. I can't remember when we last had a spider in the house since. I have learned the lesson of compassion towards other creatures and so I no longer need to be given more 'opportunities' to learn that lesson. Is being afraid of something enough justification to kill it? No, of course not. Instead, choose to live your life full of kindness and compassion to all. In this way, you will be carrying out the functions of this human form at a much higher level of spirituality.

Showing kindness to animals includes acting to help in their survival. You can make a difference to the lives of animals from your own home:

- If you witness an injustice against an animal, or if an

animal is injured in your garden, call the RSPCA (in the UK) or your local wildlife rescue center.

- Sign petitions online for action or laws to be taken or passed to prevent cruelty to animals, such as illegal hunting or raiding ospreys' nests.
- Go further and join an organization which protects animals, one which resonates with you. There are so many to choose from, such as the World Wildlife Fund (WWF), the Dogs Trust, Cats Protection (www.cats.org.uk), the RSPCA. Animals in today's world are vulnerable. We can make a positive choice to do our bit from home to offer them a greater degree of protection. Put your kindness into action!
- Keep a secluded part of your garden untidy to give a home to hedgehogs, field mice, bugs and so on. You can also buy or make a 'bug hotel.'
- Cut a small hole in your fence to allow hedgehogs to roam between gardens, and leave out a bowl of water and some food for them. Sadly the hedgehog population has declined by 30% since 2003 to less than one million.
- Plant buddleia in your garden to attract butterflies. Butterfly numbers have dropped by a quarter in the past decade. To see butterflies flitting about in our garden is good for the soul. They remind us of the transformation which we are all undertaking as we prepare to break free from our chrysalis of living in fear and negativity to emerge into a life of freedom, reborn through love and kindness!

Care of pets

Spend quality time with your pet, whether it be a goldfish, a bunny, a cat, a dog or a horse. Don't simply ignore it and read a book or watch television. Think about your initial motivation for buying a pet. Was it to ignore it? Please, interact with your pet. Have certain times during the day when you can play a game with it indoors or in the garden. This is a kindness to your pet because you are giving it not only your attention, but also your time. Imagine if the person you adored most in the world ignored you for the greater part of the day. What emotions/reactions would that stir in you? Unhappiness? Boredom? Naughtiness (attempting to get attention by any means)?

Adopt a rescue dog or cat instead of taking a puppy or kitten. Especially if you have mobility problems and are mostly housebound, it's very tiring to train a puppy. It is also a greater kindness to take on a rescue dog and give it a second chance at a happy life.

Part IV: Kindness to the Environment

Introduction

This part of the book details how to be kinder to the environment. Just think for a moment. This planet Earth has been created for us. It has the perfect air to allow us to breathe; the perfect atmosphere to protect all living things; a star at the perfect distance and intensity to sustain and nourish everything on our planet. None of this is by coincidence. It is all by design, by the Creator. We take advantage of, and luxuriate in, this perfect world and yet do we not also see it as our place to look after it?

There is a hypothesis called the Gaia Principle, first expounded in the 1700s by Scottish geologist, James Hutton, then adopted in the 1960s by the NASA scientist, James Lovelock. He studied the planets and concluded that in the same way that our bodies are made up of billions of cells all working together as one single unit, everything on Earth also works together as one single, living, self-regulating organism—all living things, the atmosphere, plants, animals, humans, climate and so on. To continue this analogy, just as our bodies have their own regulatory systems (e.g. nervous system, respiratory system), so the Earth has its own 'systems' comprising: atmosphere (air), biosphere (all lifeforms), geosphere (soil and rock) and hydrosphere (water) (source: www.scienceclarified.com). The health of the Earth depends on all these components working well in harmony. If one system is impaired or malfunctioning, it will affect all the others. There are many reasons for impairment or malfunction: ozone thinning, unbiodegradable plastics entering the food chain, fracking, draining of water tables, to name a few, of which the common denominator is the human species.

The above theory is not entirely incompatible with that

more widely accepted in spiritual circles: that the Earth is the Creator's purpose-built environment for us to play in and discover more about what it is to be human. Take this simple analogy: we watch our children in playparks, learning socially how to share, cooperate with each other, compromise, discover consequences of their choices and actions; learning mentally using cognitive processes, thinking of solutions; learning emotionally how to quell their anger, learn from the example of others, make friends etc. In the same way that we watch our children play, God watches with benevolence, hoping that we learn to share, cooperate, compromise, discover consequences of our actions, balance our emotions and so on. As regards the environment, He hopes that we learn the need to give back to the Earth in order that it may thrive for future generations.

Nature has much to teach us in its ability to regenerate and in its healing plants. We have for many years used herbs such as chamomile to aid sleep and relax muscles, feverfew to lessen the symptoms of migraine or arthritis, mint to ease symptoms of irritable bowel, and placing houseplants around the home to filter harmful pollutants from the air. The list is endless. Further, in the Shamanic tradition, each time you take from nature—for example, leaves from a healing bush, or branches from a tree to build a house or furniture—you give something back, an exchange of energy if you like. This could be a small offering of money or food perhaps. I'm not suggesting we all do this in everyday life, but we could keep this in mind as a reminder that as we *take*, so shall we *give* to the natural world. How can we give back to the environment from home? Part IV (Chapters 15–19) provides inspiration on how we can do just that in the following areas: thinking globally, acting locally; recycling/upcycling; paper usage;

food waste; organic products; the precious resource of water; the Gaia Principle; litter; and giving back to nature.

We are accustomed to taking from nature: trees to build houses and furniture; nutrients from the soil to grow food; fossil fuels to heat homes and drive cars; water for cleaning, toilets, swimming pools etc. Yet know that we can do our part to give back to nature from our armchair, and further, encourage others by our actions to do likewise. We each have our part to play in the world. We each have the capacity to change that part of the world which surrounds us by thinking globally and acting locally.

The following chapters are all interconnected and demonstrate that as we focus proactively on one area, this positively affects all the others. It is the Gaia Principle in action!

Chapter 15

Food Waste

The first way in which we can give back to the environment is through food. In the UK 18 million tonnes of food waste is generated each year (source: www.foodawarecic.org.uk), totaling around £23 billion per annum. Supermarket sell-by dates, three-for-two offers and the practice of requiring uniformly sized fruit and vegetables from suppliers all contribute to the challenge of food waste—a problem posed to the whole of society. As consumers, we often buy more food than we need. Further, the perception by many of us is that food is unsafe to eat past its *sell-by* date. However, we needn't throw out perfectly edible food just past its sell-by date. The sell-by date is a stock control mechanism and most food is perfectly fine for a few days afterwards. The exception is meat and dairy products with a use-by date. You must heed the *use-by* dates as these are given for safety reasons. Bacterial growth in these short shelf-life foods can give you very severe food poisoning if you eat them.

Where does responsibility lie in approaching the challenge of food waste—with the consumer, the retailer, the supplier, the local council, or government? The answer is all of these. Local councils are beginning to address the problem head-on by increasing food recycling and sending it to anaerobic digestion plants to generate electricity. Personal and corporate responsibility, however, also needs to play a greater part. More education in schools for the next generation is essential. Supermarkets need to loosen the requirement for uniformity of fruit and vegetables, so incurring less waste at producer level. We can also do our part. Here are some suggestions which arise from my experience:

- Only buy as much food as we will use.
- Use a grocery list and stick to it.
- Avoid impulse buys.
- Use up vegetables past their best by making soup.
- Freeze food.
- Use up leftovers.
- Donate what you won't use.
- Store food properly to avoid early deterioration.
- Use up the earliest sell-by date produce first.
- Compost wilted vegetables.
- Give thanks at every meal for the abundance of food we have.
- Write on the packaging the day you open cartons of perishables such as smoothies or humus to remind yourself of when they need to be used by. This avoids throwing out food unnecessarily.
- Resolve not to waste food.

There is another challenge which may affect us to a greater degree in coming years and decades and that is the availability of land. As populations expand worldwide, land becomes scarcer or is used to grow other crops such as oil-seed rape. One strand in the solution to this is to grow our own on what land we have. Growing our own food has risen in popularity in recent years as a reaction to the intensive farming methods used previously. Certainly, if we are able, growing some of our own produce returns an element of control to us, the consumer. This can range from sowing our own seeds, to growing herbs in a window box, to planting one or two seed potatoes in a potato bag or raised beds of our favourite vegetables in the garden. If you want to grow your own food, remember to think about possible pests and how you can control them organically. Alternatively (or additionally), buy produce from your local organic farmer's market.

We may have to be more inventive in the future in the food we eat, to include more seaweed, insects, algae and so on. On the face of it, these don't sound so appetizing. There still remains a degree of consumer disgust in the West regarding the consumption of insects. However, some people already consume spirulina algae in healthy smoothies, and seaweed is already present in foods we eat. For example, we use nori seaweed to make sushi rolls, and dulse seaweed flakes can be added to many foods to add an *umami* taste). In fact there has been a 147% increase in seaweed-flavored drinks and foods in the past four years (source: Mintel, March 2016). Please refer to the Further Reading List for further information.

These small measures we can take at home are a huge kindness to the next generation and will help to reduce the mountains of landfill waste of excess food. It is worthwhile and we can all make a difference. You may want to write to newspapers and magazines to highlight the issues of food waste if this resonates with you. If you change even one person's viewpoint or habits in terms of wasting food (even if that person is you), then you will have made a difference, so well done.

Chapter 16

Paper

In this digital age it is surprising that we still consume such a large quantity of paper in daily life. Just think, we have newspapers, magazines, mail, packaging, printer paper, wrapping paper, post-it notes, envelopes and so on. But why should we care about how much paper we use? This is because the more trees which are felled, the less CO_2 is extracted from the atmosphere, resulting in that trapped CO_2 rising and thinning the ozone layer. Remember that the ozone layer protects the Earth from the sun's rays. A thinner ozone layer means a heating up of the planet, causing more and more extremes in weather conditions all over the world.

Winter flooding and prolonged dry spells are normal events in some parts of the world, but these incidences have become more and more extreme of late, as well as increasing in frequency. For example, some parts of California have experienced a prolonged state of drought for over three years. Parts of the UK have been battered by repeated winter storms containing significantly more rainfall, resulting in severe flooding to properties and loss of life. Bangladesh is being battered by more hurricanes year on year, and destructive cyclones are wreaking environmental damage on Pacific Rim countries as well. If these environmental effects are something you would like to play a small part in extenuating, here are some examples of how to reduce paper usage from home, all of which arise from my own experience:

- Always put your paper in the correct recycling bin.

Otherwise it goes to landfill which produces methane which heats up the planet.

- Recycle magazines and books—take them to your doctor's surgery or hospital when you have an appointment, donate them to coffee shops or charity shops, or pass them on to friends.
- Order e-books and e-audiobooks to cut down on paper.

There are other, more direct ways in which you can offer your support to protecting trees. I've recently discovered through a crowdfunding website a project called ArBolivia which pays farmers in Bolivia to sustainably manage the forests in their country instead of the traditional 'slash and burn' method of cutting down trees and not replacing them. (Please refer to the Further Reading and Multimedia List at the back of the book for more details.) ArBolivia is a long-term project where expertise and materials are provided to enable the farmers to grow their own replacement trees in nurseries, to tend the existing forests and to provide wood for local wood mills and furniture manufacturers. I'm not being paid to recommend particular projects and there is a multitude to choose from. This is simply the one which resonated with me. We need to recognize that we cannot support every project, either with our time or finances, and so it is essential to choose wisely one or two projects which really fire your imagination and sing to you.

Another way to reduce paper usage is by reducing our Christmas cards list. Many of us send greetings via Facebook now. It's probably true that written cards sent by post will soon become obsolete since the current generation favors online, immediate greetings. Try sending Christmas and birthday greetings via your social media online presence. This is especially helpful for those of us who find writing to be painful or a chore. If writing Christmas cards comes under that category for you, then do yourself a kindness as well as a kindness to the trees and cut down on the amount of cards which you write and send each year.

Upcycle last year's Christmas cards. Cut out parts of the designs to use as gift tags on presents.

Buy recycled paper products, such as toilet paper, writing paper, paper vases, picture frames, Christmas tree ornaments, reusable shopping bags. Again, refer to the Further Reading and Multimedia List at the back for my recommendations.

Chapter 17

Water—Our Most Precious Resource

We should be grateful for the abundance of water we have and treasure it. It is important to cherish and appreciate our water since as the climate changes and heats up, water is becoming scarce. It may well become the most precious resource of the twenty-first century, more so than oil or gas, which are waning in popularity. It's only once we become more informed of the amount of water we waste that we can decide to what extent we need to change our habits. Knowing some of the facts may make you change your mind and act differently from now on as a kindness to the environment.

Here are just a few surprising statistics: Each person in the UK uses around 150 liters of water per day and one third of this is wasted running down the plughole or flushed down toilets. This has been rising by 1% per year since 1930. (See www.waterwise.org.uk (2011) for more details.) Did you know that a running tap uses 6 liters of water per minute? And a shower between 9 and 45 liters per minute? And finally, that toilet flushing accounts for 30% of our daily water usage?

Read this list of ways in which you can reduce your water usage from home. I'm not suggesting that you adopt each one but start slowly and build from there:

- Turn the tap off when you brush your teeth.
- Don't flush every visit to the loo. Follow the maxim: "If it's yellow, let it mellow; if it's brown, flush it down."
- Use leftover water from your night-time drinks to

water the houseplants.

- Put a water butt in your garden connected to a drainpipe and use it to wash the car, windows, water the plants etc.
- Use dishwater to water garden plants.
- If you have an old toilet, install a system-displacement device which reduces the volume of water in your flush by about 1 to 3 liters (this could be a brick placed in the cistern).
- Don't let water run away. It is a precious resource.

Becoming more informed on these environmental issues is also a kindness to yourself. Choose ones which resonate with you since if you are not interested in a topic, you will be much less inclined to take action. And do pass on your knowledge to the next generation. Go on, do something great for your environment.

We are not all meant to be eco-warriors fighting on the global stage, but we can affect the world around us. We can affect our neighborhood, our own gardens, our town and country. We can get involved in decision-making to do with issues over the climate by making our views known to local councils and government.

Another kindness is to support online global campaigns. If you cannot offer financial support to a particular cause, you may choose to share their website with your online contacts, or you can offer up good wishes or prayers for their success. Know that the power of our thoughts is paramount so make them positive and kind.

One such project I came across after seeing an advert in a *Healthy* magazine was Walk In Her Shoes, run by the charity CARE International. The aim of the charity campaign is to bring to people's attention the issue of the scarcity and inequality in access to water in some parts of

the world, in this case Ethiopia. Children, especially girls, have to walk hours to collect water each day, twice per day. This prevents girls from being educated, going to school and securing a better future for themselves. At present, they are stuck in this poverty cycle because of lack of access to water. The campaign Walk In Her Shoes takes place in March every year and involves walking the same amount of steps each day for one week as these young girls have to do to collect water, around 10,000 steps. The money raised goes towards building water wells and improving access to water to these remote villages. As an ex-teacher living in Scotland, where we are blessed with an infinite amount of water (rain!), this project resonated strongly with me.

Because I have reduced mobility and am unable to walk this amount, I had to think outside the box to come up with a plan to enable me to contribute in some way. I decided to run a Tea and Cake Morning instead, inviting friends and family. We raised double the projected target through their amazing generosity. This was then doubled again by the UK government which match-funded all amounts raised. So you see, we can make a difference from home, from our armchair! When our focus is projected outwards to others' needs, to the greater good, the kindness and generosity of spirit in our own hearts increases tenfold.

Chapter 18

Chemicals and Additives

Chemicals and additives have their uses in products, such as antimicrobial preservatives. Four such additives are parabens, SLS (sodium lauryl sulfate), limonene and microbeads. These chemicals and plastics are used in a plethora of everyday products, from cosmetics to scented candles to cleaning fluids.

In my 'previous' life (before ill health) I gave no thought to what cosmetics contained or to which preservatives were in cleaning products etc. Fibromyalgia has been a blessing in many ways, including an increased hypersensitivity to many things—chief among these: chemicals. Itchy skin after showering, facial rashes after shampooing, wheezing after using antibacterial sprays and so on. Physical symptoms are the outer display of inner unease and so I am grateful for them in highlighting this issue for me. Hypersensitivity was the principal reason for my gradual change to organic products. However, for some people it may be ethical. For others still, they will be happy to maintain the status quo. We each have to make our own choices and these will be individual and distinct. Further, none of us should judge another on the basis of their choices.

The use of gentler products, and preferably organic, means that there will have been no harmful fertilizers used in the production of the ingredients, which is better for the environment and for ourselves. The four main additives in products which I would urge caution in using are, as mentioned above: parabens, SLS, limonene and microbeads. There is no need to purchase products

containing these ingredients since there are many products which are free from parabens or sodium lauryl sulfate, as well as a wealth of cruelty-free products not tested on animals. Health-food shops and online companies are a good place to start (see the Further Reading and Multimedia List for my recommendations). Vouchers for natural, ethical companies make thoughtful birthday and Christmas gifts as a way to gently bring these issues to the attention of your loved ones.

Parabens, SLS, limonene and microbeads

Parabens are chemicals which are added to foods and to some cosmetic products such as underarm deodorants, primarily as preservatives to prevent bacterial growth. They are xeno-estrogens (they mimic estrogen in the body). It has long been feared that xeno-estrogens may affect the reproductive systems of male mammals. The effect of parabens on human and marine biology has been researched in scientific studies on both sides of the argument. One such study (see P. D. Darbre, in *Journal of Applied Toxicology*, 2004) revealed parabens present in biopsy samples from breast tumors. Further, a study in September 2015 showed that eight species of marine mammals around the coasts of the USA had synthetic parabens stored in their tissue (source: ACS Environmental Science and Technology). On the basis of this study, it would seem that parabens are finding their way to our oceans and into marine mammals. Further study will be needed to establish what effects this may have on marine life. Obviously there will be research which returns opposite findings. We each have to make up our own minds. I choose to avoid parabens.

SLS (sodium lauryl sulfate), used as a foaming agent, is also xeno-estrogenic and strips the skin of natural oils. SLS

can cause skin and eye irritation and, like many chemicals, is also tested on animals. SLS is absorbed into the body via the skin and it can mimic the effects of estrogen in the body (source: www.livestrong.com), which may have future health implications for humans. For me personally, this is an unnecessary chemical and one to be avoided.

Limonene is present in many cleaning products and scented candles and in itself is not harmful. When it comes into contact with ozone in the air, every two of its molecules forms one molecule of formaldehyde which is a known human carcinogen (source: National Centre for Atmospheric Science, University of York, in conjunction with the British television program *Trust Me, I'm a Doctor*, January 2016). Opening the window when burning candles is advisable, as is placing houseplants, especially ivy, geranium, lavender and fern, near scented candles to absorb the formaldehyde. Please do more research and come to your own decision on this issue. For me, I choose to err on the side of caution and use unscented candles or natural incense instead.

Microbeads are used in face creams and washes as exfoliators. These tiny plastic beads can't be filtered by our water systems so end up in rivers and seas, swallowed by fish and ultimately passed along the marine food-chain back to us. If you want to learn more about their use, visit: www.beatthemicrobead.org. They are not biodegradable and are impossible to remove. Consumers are largely unaware of their presence in their cosmetics. If you are concerned about microbeads, there is an app which reads the barcode of a product and indicates if it contains microbeads. This puts control back into consumer hands to make an informed choice before purchase. Further, 82 NGOs (non-governmental organizations) from over 35 countries are supporting the campaign to ban the

microbead (as at March 2016). Go online and register your
support!

Chapter 19

Litter and Upcycling

You must treat the Earth well. It was not given to you by your parents. It is loaned to you by your children.
Kikuyu Kenyan proverb

Litter

Littering is, in my view, the outward manifestation of an inner lack of respect, for the self, for others, for the animal kingdom and for the environment. There are many in society who have become so separate from each other that littering is viewed as a 'right,' and the task of clearing it up the responsibility of others. We live on this planet as if we have another one to go to. Councils, governments, public institutions all do their part in tackling the blight of littering, but funding pressures mean budgets are often spent on 'more essential' services. On a positive note, local volunteer groups regularly organize litter clean-ups in many towns. All of these establishments have people at their core, and it is people who will need to change their habits of thinking and behavior, as individuals in their own homes, gardens, streets and neighborhoods, if littering is to be addressed successfully.

Care for our part of the world over which we can effect change is easier than we might think, as is leading by example and having higher expectations of everyone in society, from young to old, to look after our world. For we do not have another world to go to. We are on Earth to learn what it is to be human. Is thoughtlessness an essential part of the human make-up? Of course not, but many of us are wrapped up in the ego's false ideas about life: that it is

our right to take whatever we want for ourselves; that we can forgo any responsibilities which are unpalatable to us.

And yet there are two sides to a coin which if tossed would reveal heads as our rights and tails as our responsibilities. We cannot have one without the other if we are to maintain a caring and successful society. A shift in our gaze outwards to the greater good of others is needed. How can we change our habits on litter from the comfort of our armchair?

We must teach our children to dispose of litter responsibly. If children see adults dropping litter with no thought of any consequences, then the younger generation may assume that this is acceptable behavior. Parents are the primary educators of their children, but an active partnership with schools to teach children social responsibility is also vital.

Make sure that you recycle well in the home. It only takes a few minutes to do this each day and get into the routine. It is not solely the younger generation who need to be encouraged to do this. Many older people can also be affected by malaise, apathy or a sense of non-commitment.

Keep your home tidy. Our homes are an echo of our inner emotions, so make sure your home is tidy with no dirty dishes lying around or overflowing rubbish bins. A messy home environment tells you and others that you are not interested in your surroundings, your home, even yourself. Pick up litter thrown or blown into your garden; tidy up your kitchen and bathroom especially, as germs can flourish here; do your own bit to try and improve the mini environment around you. Lead by example.

Housework. Know that when you clean and tidy your home an added benefit is that you cleanse your own energy field, since dirt and rubbish lying around can drain you of energy. Some of us are unable to do housework. Could you do a kindness to a young person and offer them this job as paid work experience? Do you receive disability or other benefits/income which might be used towards this cost? Remember, do not see problems; think how you might solve them.

Declutter. An accumulation of possessions speaks to me of inner chaos, an inability to make decisions. This indicates that we are stuck on our life path, not wanting to 'throw out' the past in case we need it for the future. Yet the road to happiness is through the present. Here are some ideas of how to declutter:

- In this digital age, there is no need to keep past copies of professional journals or old coursework books from our college days 30 years prior. Throw out the journals and even the books, as students access information digitally now.
- Throw out old broken furniture which cannot be repaired or donated. Local councils (in the UK) will collect this for you on request.
- Donate clothes which no longer fit you. A good benchmark: If you haven't worn them for a year, it's time to let them go. There are various charities which collect unwanted clothes from your doorstep, or you could ask someone to donate them to a local charity shop in town if you have mobility issues.
- Go through your old photograph albums and throw out all but a few essential ones, or scan some of these to save as digital files on your computer. Photograph